AFTA SpringerBriefs in Family Therapy

Series Editor

Carmen Knudson-Martin
Education & Counseling, Rogers Hall
Lewis & Clark Grad Sch
Portland, OR, USA

SpringerBriefs present concise summaries of cutting-edge research and practical applications. Featuring compact volumes of 50 to 125 pages, the series covers a range of content from professional to academic. Typical topics might include: A timely report of state-of-the art analytical techniques A bridge between new research results, as published in journal articles, and a contextual literature review A snapshot of a hot or emerging topic An in-depth case study or clinical example A presentation of core concepts that students must understand in order to make independent contributions

More information about this series at http://www.springer.com/series/11846

Karen Mui-Teng Quek • Alexander Lin Hsieh
Editors

Intersectionality in Family Therapy Leadership

Professional Power, Personal Identities

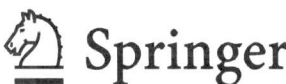 Springer

Editors
Karen Mui-Teng Quek
Marriage and Family Therapy Program
Biola University (Talbot School of Theology)
La Mirada, CA, USA

Alexander Lin Hsieh
Couple and Family Therapy Program
Alliant International University
Sacramento, CA, USA

ISSN 2196-5528 ISSN 2196-5536 (electronic)
AFTA SpringerBriefs in Family Therapy
ISBN 978-3-030-67976-7 ISBN 978-3-030-67977-4 (eBook)
https://doi.org/10.1007/978-3-030-67977-4

This Springer imprint is published by the registered company Springer Nature Switzerland AG
The registered company address is: Gewerbestrasse 11, 6330 Cham, Switzerland

Series Foreword

AFTA Springer Briefs in Family Therapy is an official publication of the American Family Therapy Academy. Each volume focuses on the practice and policy implications of innovative systemic research and theory in family therapy and allied fields. Our goal is to make information about families and systemic practices in societal contexts widely accessible in a reader friendly, conversational, and practical style. AFTA's core commitment to equality, social responsibility, and justice are represented in each volume.

Discussions of how to address the power inherent in leadership positions almost invariably speak as though leaders represent the dominant culture. In *Intersectionality in Family Therapy Leadership—Professional Power, Personal Identities,* editors Karen Quek and Alexander Hsieh offer a collection of highly personal accounts of holding positions of power in family therapy supervision, education, and administration while themselves also inhabiting marginalized social identities. The willingness of the authors to reflect on these complex intersections and share their stories is a true gift to the field. Persons holding marginalized identities will find models to whom they can relate and will be inspired to examine their own intersectionalities. Persons holding dominant culture privilege will gain insight regarding their colleagues' experiences managing highly nuanced positions of power while also invisible and discriminated against.

By bringing their stories to the foreground, the authors take a step toward dismantling taken-for-granted assumptions regarding how leadership is/should be enacted and performed. They open space for multiple challenges and opportunities in how leadership in family therapy and related disciplines is envisioned. Their work will be welcomed by many, but especially by new generations of leaders from diverse backgrounds who follow their lead. With gratitude and respect to the authors on behalf of the American Family Therapy Academy, I invite you to enter their multifaceted worlds.

AFTA Springer Briefs in Family Therapy   Carmen Knudson-Martin
Lewis & Clark College
Portland, OR, USA

AFTA Springer Briefs in Family Therapy

A publication of the American Family Therapy Academy

Founded in 1977, the **American Family Therapy Academy** is a nonprofit organization of leading family therapy teachers, clinicians, program directors, policymakers, researchers, and social scientists dedicated to advancing systemic thinking and practices for families in their social context.

Vision

AFTA envisions a just world by transforming social contexts that promote health, safety, and well-being of all families and communities.

Mission

AFTA's mission is developing, researching, teaching, and disseminating progressive, just family therapy and family-centered practices and policies.

Acknowledgments

Intersectionality in Family Therapy Leadership—Professional Power, Personal Identities is about the Marriage and Family Therapy educators' collective encountering of inequality and discrimination as a result of our social locations as well as our greater access to power and resources that we used in initiating social change within our sphere of influence. With collective action through sharing experiences with colleagues, we begin to gain some successes in our professional work.

The publication of this book would not have been possible without the exceptional support of Carmen Knudson-Martin, the Series Editor of AFTA Spring Briefs in Family Therapy. We are grateful to Carmen who gave us this amazing opportunity to tell our stories about professional power and achievement on the one hand and stories of discrimination experienced in higher education and clinical environment on the other. We are thankful for her editorial skill, her competency in subject matter, and her open and analytical critiques that have helped shape this book. Her help has been invaluable to all of us.

Our special thanks go to the authors who have contributed to this book: Hao-Min Chen, Ph.D., Texas A&M University, Central Texas, TX; Christie Eppler, Ph.D., Seattle University, Seattle, WA; Sergio Pereyra, Ph.D., Fresno State University, Fresno, CA; Gita Seshadri, Ph.D., Alliant International University, Sacramento, CA; and Narumi Tanaguchi, Ph.D., University of Winnipeg, Manitoba, Canada. We appreciate the authors' transparency about their cultural journeys. Each chapter deconstructs biases in systems and relational dynamics, which is critical to growth and healing. By bravely sharing their personal stories, the authors give voice to the process of navigating the challenges of uncertainty, frustration, confusion, fear, and inner tension.

We also extend our heartfelt thanks to Natalie Kwan and Rosa Nam, our grammar gurus for many hours of reading and editing drafts of the chapters. We appreciate their commitment to literary excellence. Thanks to the American Family Therapy Academy for promoting multi-voiced scholarship and to Judy Jones and the team at Springer for overseeing the publication of this project.

Karen Mui-Teng Quek
Alexander Lin Hsieh

Contents

About the Editors

Karen Mui-Teng Quek is Professor and Program Director of Marriage and Family Therapy at Biola University's Talbot School of Theology, La Mirada, CA. Her research interest in the development of a healthy professional identity examines the intersection of multiple social locations (e.g., race, ethnicity, gender, etc.) and workplace leadership. Karen has published a number of articles on cross-cultural competency in clinical supervision and couples relational dynamic. She co-edited *Transition and Change in Collectivist Family Life: Strategies for Clinical Practice with Asian Americans* (2017), Springer Series in Family Therapy.

Alexander Lin Hsieh is a core faculty member and Clinical Training Coordinator for Alliant International University's CSPP Couple and Family Therapy program in Sacramento, and Program Director for the online campus. He has conducted empirical research on adolescent depression and shame. Additionally, he conducts research on cultural competency, sex therapy and sex addictions, inclusion in academics, minority issues, and Asian-American families and couples in therapy. He regularly works clinically with interracial couples, Asian-American families, pornography and sex addictions, and adolescents.

Contributors

Hao-Min Chen Marriage and Family Therapy Program, Texas A & M University-Central Texas, Killeen, TX, USA

Christie Eppler Couples and Family Therapy, Seattle University, Seattle, WA, USA

Alexander Lin Hsieh Couple and Family Therapy Program, Alliant International University, Sacramento, CA, USA

Sergio B. Pereyra Marriage and Family Therapy Program, Fresno State University, Fresno, CA, USA

Karen Mui-Teng Quek Marriage and Family Therapy Program, Biola University (Talbot School of Theology), La Mirada, CA, USA

Gita Seshadri Couple and Family Therapy Program, Alliant International University, Sacramento, CA, USA

Narumi Taniguchi Master of Marriage and Family Therapy Program, The University of Winnipeg, Winnipeg, MB, Canada

Chapter 1
Introduction: Our Contexts and Frameworks

Reflections on race/ethnicity, gender, and cultural experiences are important because they inform the experiences of current and future mental health professionals. *Intersectionality in Family Therapy Leadership—Professional Power, Personal Identities* is a compilation of marital and family educators' socially located narratives. This is a timely book because it affords an opportunity for training institutions and individual therapists to consider personalized accounts of discrimination and encounters with transforming oppressive systems for inclusion and equality. Themes of culture, gender, spirituality, connection, power, oppression, and resilience are woven throughout each story.

We appreciate the authors' transparency about their cultural journeys, including recognizing their critical experiences of subjugation and privilege. Each chapter deconstructs biases in systems and relational dynamics, which is critical to growth and healing. To analyze personal experience is no easy task, as it requires deep self-reflection and vulnerability. By bravely sharing their personal stories, the authors give voice to how many navigate the challenges of uncertainty, frustration, confusion, fear, and inner tension. The authors articulate the tensions between confronting injustice and creating formative spaces where communities flourish. We also want to highlight that the time between when the authors first sat out to write their narratives to the completion of this book, the social context has dramatically changed. The timeline included a global pandemic, rise in social justice unrest, and a dramatic transformation of many education systems from on-ground education to virtual education. While the social context continues to shift, the internal processing of each author will continue to develop. This is the work of dismantling oppressive systems.

© Springer Nature Switzerland AG 2021
K. M.-T. Quek, A. L. Hsieh (eds.), *Intersectionality in Family Therapy Leadership*, AFTA SpringerBriefs in Family Therapy,
https://doi.org/10.1007/978-3-030-67977-4_1

By combining the theory of intersectionality with autoethnography, the chapters underline the multiplicity of socially located conflicts inherent in the daily lives of faculty of color and their allies. Additional frameworks, including the Latina/o critical race theory, an eco-developmental and the postmodern lenses, support storylines that illustrate commitment to social justice and respect the local social and cultural patterns. Privileged and marginalized identities undoubtedly affect not only pedagogical choices and administrative styles, but also the perceptions of colleagues, staff, and students. These narratives consider the ways in which oppression and privilege have been woven into systemic therapy's larger systems, therapists' own relational patterns, and interactions with clients.

In recounting our experiences, the authors employ intersectionality and autoethnography to attend to cultural and social contexts and processes, acknowledging our continuous subjection to gendered, ethnic and racial inequality in the profession and the larger system, as well as constructing solutions to the collective systemic challenge.

Theory of intersectionality describes the need to explore social locations, how they interact, and how systemic interactions produce experiences of marginalization, power, and stigma (Crenshaw, 1989; Shields, 2008). Just and equitable administration and pedagogy require regular examination of social location in terms of impact on leadership, learning, privilege, invisibility, bias, and assumptions (Few-Demo, 2014). The chapters explore how do the authors' presence at administrative meetings and in the classroom alter the environment.

Theory of autoethnography connects the self to the social spaces by telling our relational and institutional stories in order to recover a marginalized and self-reflective gap (Ellis & Bochner, 2000). It sheds light on diverse social location as it moves through particular contexts. Simultaneously, autoethnography allows for the narrators to deconstruct contradictory and competing tensions within as they connect the personal self to the social context. This has given voice to silenced tensions that lie underneath observable behaviors in their narratives.

Social location refers to the social position a person occupies within a particular society and culture, and is based upon social properties deemed to be important by any given society. Our social location may fall under different categories of race, gender, age, religion, socioeconomic status, and sexual orientation (Crenshaw, 1989). Societal and cultural norms heavily influence our social standing. While many locations are visible, the lesser known ones, such as generational influences, natural origin, education, and ability, are hidden (Hays, 2001). We explore systems of power within the diversity of social locations that create experiences of privilege and disadvantage, depending upon the different social positions we occupy.

Privilege refers to unearned access to resources and social power that are only available to some as a result of their advantaged social group membership (Adams, Bell, & Griffin, 2007). The professional roles of clinician, supervisor, professor, and program director are automatically granted power and privilege by their title because they symbolize authority and expertise.

In the following accounts, the authors ask themselves: How do administrators, colleagues, staff, and students respond to us based on our differing social identities?

How do we perpetuate the academy's system of privilege? What role does culture play when communicating? How is it possible to unpack invisible privilege? How do we promote systemic change and succeed in an academic career path?

The purpose of this collection is to illuminate diverse life stories from authors who thrived within multiple contexts. The text prioritizes voices of authors who reside in marginalized social location, which is critical, as these accounts have often been ignored, subjected, and silenced. The text also includes accounts of the responsible use of privilege to actively practice and support social justice which is significant for positive change. Our intent is to provide a contemporary perspective of how accomplished marriage and family therapists/educators awakened to their culturally situated selves and found resilience. May readers find comfort, challenge, and inspiration within these accounts.

References

Adams, M., Bell, L. A., & Griffin, P. (Eds.). (2007). *Teaching for diversity and social justice* (2nd ed.). New York, NY: Routledge.

Crenshaw, K. (1989). Demarginalizing the intersection of race and sex: A black feminist critique of antidiscrimination doctrine, feminist theory and antiracist politics. *University of Chicago Legal Forum, 1989.*

Ellis, C., & Bochner, A. P. (2000). Autoethnography, personal narrative, reflexivity. In N. K. Denzin & Y. S. Lincoln (Eds.), *Handbook of qualitative research* (2nd ed., pp. 733–768). Thousand Oaks, CA: Sage.

Few-Demo, A. L. (2014). Intersectionality as the "new" critical approach in feminist family studies: Evolving racial/ethnic feminisms and critical race theories. *Journal of Family Theory & Review, 6*(2), 169–183.

Hays, P. A. (2001). *Addressing cultural complexities in practice: A framework for clinicians and counselors.* Washington, DC: American Psychological Association.

Shields, S. A. (2008). Gender: An intersectionality perspective. *Sex Roles, 59,* 302–311.

Chapter 2
Intersecting Stories of Power and Discrimination: Narrative of a Female Program Director of Color

Karen Mui-Teng Quek

As a female faculty of color, I am no stranger to discrimination on the job. But many incidents are not overt, making it hard to interpret, label, and talk about my experiences. Since I do not often give voice to my feelings of being discriminated against, I do not tend to describe myself as being subjected to gender, racial, or ethnic discrimination. Nonetheless, it is there and it is subtle (Sue et al., 2011).

Here is one story that describes less overt discrimination in all of its ugliness: When I worked as the program director at a university, two students made academic requests to switch programs. I should have been the final decision maker on such matters, but an administrative officer approved the students' requests without consulting me. I did not learn about these changes until a year later when the students were registering for classes. Because the administrator had since resigned by that time, I was left to salvage the situation. I had to explain to these students that the approval they had received previously was in fact invalid because it had not been rendered in accordance with university policy and procedures, and I had to attend to their resultant frustration about the system.

This was one of several occasions when I had been excluded from a programmatic decision-making process by this administrator. Though we had a cordial working relationship, this pattern of bypassing me made me uneasy. Many times I felt the need to give her face and to tolerate her behavior because of who she was in relation to me—she was an older White female who had been in her position for almost 20years. She carried privilege as to race, age, and seniority at work because I was a faculty of color, younger than her, and new to the institution. In this particular situation, she left behind a systemic problem for everyone to resolve. But I was also left wondering, "Was this done to undermine my authority? Or was it an

K. M.-T. Quek (✉)
Marriage and Family Therapy Program, Biola University (Talbot School of Theology),
La Mirada, CA, USA
e-mail: karen.quek@biola.edu

© Springer Nature Switzerland AG 2021
K. M.-T. Quek, A. L. Hsieh (eds.), *Intersectionality in Family Therapy Leadership*, AFTA SpringerBriefs in Family Therapy,
https://doi.org/10.1007/978-3-030-67977-4_2

oversight?" It was difficult to articulate this experience because the discrimination was subtle and invisible, but also persistent, as I had experienced many other similar incidents with her. Research has shown that professional experiences like this involving gender, ethnic, and racial discrimination are common among Asians, Hispanics, and Blacks (Turner, 2002).

Before I left Singapore to study in the United States many years ago, a wise pastor said to me, "Be yourself." I took this to mean that I should be true to who I am. I am a Christian. I am a cis-female. I am a Singaporean of Chinese descent. These social identities intersect and inform one another. This combination of gender, ethnicity, and race categorizes me as a woman of color. My social location in the US context also includes an added layer of being a migrant.

As an immigrant woman of color, I may find strength and power in my ethnicity, gender, and national status. A colleague used to say that I am comfortable in my own skin, but my challenge is being a woman of color in a dominant discourse that privileges a particular race, gender, sexual orientation, religion, and national status. In this way, the Asian female's journey of becoming and being a mid-level faculty leader reflects the complexities of the current landscape of academia and the multiple hierarchies that female faculty of color must contend with. Over time, I have learned to develop my sense of self from different social locations and make meaning of contradictory experiences of power and disadvantage. This chapter is, therefore, a self-reflection that explores my professional experiences and situates my narrative within a particular cultural and social context. Specifically, it is the story of one female educator of color in leadership examining the factors that shape her professionally.

I am now a faculty member and program director of a marriage and family therapy (MFT) program. My current work focuses on the overall operation of the MFT program, including oversight of the curriculum and of clinical training. Having worked in higher education institutions for more than a decade, I would say that ethnicity, gender, immigrant status, and religion are deeply intertwined with teaching and research agendas, mentorship goals, and the leadership style I employ to navigate the MFT program. My identity as an Asian female academic leader cannot be split neatly into any one of these characterizations, as they are intertwined and visible. What is not visible is my religion and its impact on my professional life. While my Christian faith in the Protestant tradition is privileged in American culture, my gender and racial and ethnic backgrounds are not. For example, female faculty of color tend to be undervalued in academia, prompting a higher rate of attrition and lower rates of tenure advancement (Ponjuan, Conley, & Trower, 2011). In general, Asian Americans experience their fair share of racism and discrimination (Wong & Halgin, 2006). Recent reports of microaggressions, racial profiling, xenophobia, hate incidents, hate crimes, and harassment toward Asian Americans and Pacific Islanders during the COVID-19 pandemic are prime examples (Raukko, 2020).

Reflecting on where I fit within these systems of advantage and disadvantage in higher education is as uncomfortable as it is necessary. Being uncomfortable in this manner may be key in today's world because navigating the tension between the dominant discourse about professional work and the discourse on power and disadvantage with its emphasis on gendered and racialized groups can be emotionally exhausting. Truth be told, as a faculty member in a leadership role, I often find myself struggling to manage a particular set of interpersonal and complex professional spaces within the institutions I work. But to be able to weave past and present experiences and future plans into a compelling whole is necessary and generative, which is why I am sharing my personal experiences. As is customary, I assigned pseudonyms and altered details to protect identities of others in these narratives.

Starting My Academic Journey

I started my academic journey during the new millennium. The transition to a new working life in academe was refreshing after many years working at several non-profit corporations in Singapore and in the United States. I entered academe with life experiences, confidence, and excitement. This shift was a continuation of my life goal, which is to foster loving and healthy couple and family relationships that promote mental health. Because of this end, I am committed to the training of marriage and family therapists—not only practical techniques, but also developing the selfhood of therapists. However, teaching is not all I do; advancing to an administrative position seemed to be the next logical step. As I took on a program director position, I became more aware of the multiple forms of hierarchy that underlie institutions of higher education. I have worked with several universities, and moving from one school to the next taught me how to adapt and be flexible in new environments. As I encountered diverse academic cultures, I learned about and came to appreciate many academic structures. But I also experienced and observed cultural bias and insensitivities. I found myself in many painful situations of holding a position that is simultaneously privileged and disadvantaged.

In reflecting on my narratives, I choose to enter, not escape, the tangles of teaching and administering an MFT program. Over the years, I had subconsciously written off many negative experiences for various reasons. I do not like to make people feel uncomfortable, whether individually or as a group. The mental strain associated with trying to manage such tensions may be too much to bear. I do not know how to confront the issues, as these are not so clear-cut. Many colleagues who did confront them did so as a last straw before they left. While my experiences are not generalizable to all female faculty of color, this reflective account provides important tools for other professionals in similar situations.

The call for cross-cultural competence in academic institutions has not translated into an equitable work environment for faculty of color in leadership. Interpersonal and professional challenges have inhibited the development of such leaders. Many faculty leaders of color have encountered obstacles related to the intersectionality of their ethnicity, race, gender, and immigrant status. For decades, faculty leaders of color have narrated their experiences of isolation and harassment (Stanley, 2006), exposing the scars that result when colleagues question their competence and achievements or even backstab them (Chang, Longman, & Franco, 2014). Scholars of color have also documented experiences with professional jealousy and unsupportive supervisors, difficulties in career advancement, experiences of hostility, microaggressions, and treatment as outsiders (Griffin & Reddick, 2011; Harris, Trepal, Prado, & Robinson, 2019; Lumby & Coleman, 2007; Stanley, 2006).

These sentiments echo my own experiences; I am not alone. More often than not, faculty leaders of color seem to get the short end of the stick in an already-difficult field. Like many others, I was the only faculty member of color in the departments I have worked at. And being in administrative leadership at a programmatic level increases loneliness and isolation. I have not been trained to manage these types of challenges, and thus feel unprepared for them.

A Story of Discrimination: The Content

The following account is a personal example of how multiple social locations shaped my response to a situation of marginality.

At one university, I was the only female Asian faculty in the department. I was not happy in this role because of problems in the department, but I was also seemingly on a course toward tenure and promotion because I have a very good track record in teaching, scholarship, and service. One day, I requested to meet with the dean concerning a job offer I received from another institution. I had been agonizing for months about whether to stay or to move on, and this job offer would have been a great opportunity to get a new start. He was shocked and expressed disbelief that there were problems in the department. But instead of addressing my concerns, the dean directed me to talk to my supervisor. When I did, I was blasted for surprising her with an offer letter from another institution. While I was very surprised by the reactions of these administrators, I wanted to work on these issues rather than ignore them.

Responses of my colleagues from different institutions varied. In general, my White colleagues said that I should leave and not deal with the issues. However, my Asian American colleagues said to confront them and deal with them for the sake of the next generation. One Asian American senior colleague and a sought-after activist once remarked, "As the Chinese saying goes, be like water—water is soft, yielding, and fluid. Water wears away rock, which is rigid and unyielding" (personal conversation). As a rule, she said, if you learn to be flexible, gentle, and yielding, you will overcome whatever is rigid and hard. Harmonious working relationships are important to me as an Asian and a Christian because they embody well-being, justice, and love. Convinced that it was better to work things out, I decided to stay. I declined the new offer and stayed, thinking that I could make change happen. But there was little movement, and conversations became awkward. I felt as if I had fallen off the edge of a cliff. I second-guessed myself, and that affected my confidence. After 1 year, it became clear that I needed to move on, so I left.

Through trial and error, I learned to manage my emotions, be at peace when I do not see light at the end of the tunnel, and pick my battles carefully. There are now times when I allow negative experiences to roll off me like water off a duck's back. I look back over my academic career and realize that holding fast to my own values and beliefs based on the intersection of ethnicity, gender, and religion, while also attempting to remain objective, can be exhausting. I have had to learn which battles are worth the energy it takes to pursue them.

This situation might have ended negatively for me had there not been new insights emerging from deeper knowledge of my social location that I could draw on to help advance my passion for the MFT field. Increased self-awareness has been beneficial—I can understand myself and others better and negotiate situations and relationships with more grace, not only to guard my own spirit, but also to serve my students and the program well.

A Story of Discrimination: The Process—My Internal Dialogue

Making sense of discrimination narratives is a personal endeavor that draws on social location reflecting both a dilemma and a solution to it. It involves a dilemma because no matter how a female faculty of color responds to bias, her actions risk penalty, and her career may be obstructed (Turner, 2002). A solution can become evident when the process partially dismantles the taken-for-granted dominant discourse. When trying to make sense of my own experiences, struggles with the limits of social location can constrain my desire to vocalize my stories in ways that make me self-conscious about what I may be saying. However, Nash (2008) highlights the usefulness of considering the agency that different social locations permit in different contexts. Knowing how positions of privilege and disadvantage intersect guides me in my decision about whether to speak out and how best to describe my encounter. The more I become aware and the more I listen and try to understand others' experiences and narratives, the more I recognize the humanity in each person.

When the above incident happened, I spent much time deliberating about whether I should bring it up to my supervisor, whether the person was just ignorant, and whether it was culturally appropriate for a junior faculty member to raise such an issue. I feared what the outcome might be. I wondered how much I wanted to risk and how it would affect me and come back to haunt me. In addition to thinking about personal consequences, I also thought about the systemic impact and the others involved. How could I have broached such a sensitive subject in a way that did not cause my colleagues to feel attacked or to respond by being defensive? Risk-taking is not in my DNA in such situations. As with many such events, I swept it under the rug. Over time, however, it became a small but persistent frustration. In other similar situations, whether I moved ahead with confronting the issue or let it go, each decision carried significant consequences—draining my emotional energy and detracting from my mental health. Unfortunately, I built a tension internally. It was difficult to raise awareness about racial prejudice when White colleagues from the dominant discourse did not see power, privilege, and disadvantage, I began to rationalize that they nevertheless meant well. It would be difficult and taxing for them to perceive something from another's point of view and to do it correctly. Yes, I found myself needing to take care and protect my White colleagues from having to deal with such challenges.

Certainly, my perspective on such encounters was very much colored by my social location and the way intersectionality framed those experiences. For example, my Christian faith gives me privilege in a faith-based institution; my gender, race, and ethnicity marginalize me; and my immigration status remains hidden. Knowing how these positions of privilege and disadvantage intersect guides me in my decision to speak out and how best to describe my point. But the colliding dynamics of several social locations—racial and ethnic cultural background, female, and conservative Christian—could prove to be a "triple whammy" in processing localized discrimination. Context and locale matter. Would vocalizing my concern backfire? To not vocalize it seems cowardly and perpetuates the stereotype that Asian females are quiet and submissive. In some situations, I gave in to Asian female stereotypes by being silent, living harmoniously, and keeping the peace. Because I am already a minority in dominant spaces, it can be hard to call out situations involving a social hierarchy that lends itself to Asian female leaders being silenced. Other times, it seems the best option is to "let go and let God"—a strategy that I used in situations when I sought to practice gratitude in the midst of injustice and to pursue justice, mercy, and understanding. But how would this strategy be helpful? This sort of back-and-forth internal dialogue is critical for self-regulation, self-reflection, and processing purposes (Morin, Duhnych, & Racy, 2018).

On the one hand, the back-and-forth internal reaction may align with my personal desire to create spaces to build and engage in more conversations. On the other hand, my response was a matter of searching within myself for some principles to guide my actions. But I encountered a sense of isolation when dealing with my experiences of discrimination. A story about discrimination is not so easily integrated in my professional identity because this recognizes a subjugated identity, which Hardy (2018) remarked is constantly under assault and, therefore, needed to be protected.

Consequences Being in the Minority at Work

There is a lack of professional role models of color in academia, and even less diversity among educators in leadership roles (Moore, 2017; Stanley, 2006). Lacking mentors who possess knowledge of the minority experience means faculty of color will suffer from little sponsorship and greater feelings of isolation. Dealing with isolation and the frustration associated with trying to live up to a professional ideal that fails to support diversity is emotionally draining. These feelings can often be overwhelming. Colleagues of color have remarked that such emotions are not always visible and may instead brew in silence. There is concern that verbalizing such issues makes one appear overly sensitive, but the other option—remaining silent—has the effect of minimizing the problem. This is a constant dilemma for faculty of color.

Aside from not seeing professional role models of color, there are real costs when one is consistently in the racial and/or ethnic minority at work. Scholars have documented that faculty leaders of color may continue to face challenges in developing collegiality and may be ignored (Alexander Jr & Moore, 2008). Phillips, Rothbard, and Dumas (2009) suggest that working in isolation creates "status distance"—that is, how far one is from the institution's norm and power structure. Faculty leaders of color may share the same level of status as other colleagues at the institution, and thus should in theory have similarly high-quality relationships with those in authority. However, status distance resulting from working *in silos* often affects participation rates during discussion as well as the degree of influence one has over group decisions.

Faculty leaders of color must actively seek new ways to engage with issues around ethnicity, gender, and immigration status; develop safe spaces for deeper dialogues; and look for different resources. When we remember that we are not alone—that many came before us and many will come after us—it helps to build strength and offer respite as we navigate our individual, social, and professional environments. In the following section, I will focus more on practical ways to consider power, resources, strength, and connection within the context of academia.

Supportive Practices

Mentors Who "Get Us"

Faculty leaders of color need mentors who "get us and are not threatened by us" (Chang et al., 2014). Because of the lack of professional role models of color, having a mentor is very important. Mentors can serve as power brokers to help their mentees access opportunities within a professional network of power and privilege (Eby & Allen, 2008). My mentors have certainly helped me navigate the complex process of negotiating academic demands to ensure success in my work. I relied on both formal, traditional one-on-one mentoring, and an informal mentoring network consisting of like-minded professionals to survive and thrive in my career.

When I started my first full-time academic position, I had no prior knowledge about the benefits of mentoring. Formal mentoring was provided to me; this arrangement involved meeting regularly and having meals together, the ultimate purpose being to facilitate my adjustment to the new environment. I gained new knowledge about the culture of the university, teaching tips, advice on what to look out for, etc. Not having to seek out my own mentor was helpful. The formal mentoring was beneficial, especially since it came from someone who was from a different discipline and who was more senior. However, though this mentoring arrangement served its purpose well, it was also short-lived, limited to one semester.

Having a network of peer mentors is equally if not more important than receiving formal one-on-one mentoring, especially in the field of marriage and family sciences. This type of mentoring provides the sociopolitical capital needed to advance professionally and valuable psychosocial support in the workplace. Colleagues in my personal network mostly hail from within my discipline in MFT. I have had the especially good fortune of experiencing a student-faculty relationship evolve into a collegial relationship with my dissertation chair. She is fully aware of her social standing as a White female academic and author. She leads me into the world of academia and walks alongside me—extending opportunities to coauthor several articles, conference presentations, and scholarly publications. Clearly, she is a model to me. The connection with her throughout my PhD program and later as a colleague in a larger context is a gift. She has selflessly offered her time and words of wisdom. I can reach out to her anytime without hesitation—that is how approachable she is to me and many colleagues of color. She strongly encourages me to pursue the MFT field. And the more I learn about the relational and systemic paradigm of MFT work, the more I realize my desire to contribute to this area because the field fits my philosophical and spiritual commitment.

Additionally, a group of Asian American professors from various universities took me in as one of their own during a National Council of Family Relations annual conference I attended. Since then, we have participated in informal reciprocal support circles. I believe what brought us together was a set of shared values around care for one another, collaboration surrounding journeys of underrepresented Asian American professors, and deeper dialogue as to diversity issues. I believe this need for alliances and coalitions to connect on issues is still important to many faculty leaders of color. This is consistent with Stanley's (2006) conclusion that female educators of color seek out relationships in "safe spaces"—professional and personal mentoring outside of their own institutions.

Tap into Resources Wisely

Being the only female Asian faculty member in my program, I was able to gain a little more funding to advance my scholarship. Therefore, I have attended more conferences and shared my research trajectory in various academic spaces. This support was helpful in that I gained more exposure for my work and was able to raise my scholarship voice and visibility. Positional power as a resource is definitely available to me because of my role as a faculty member and a program leader. Seeking ways to redistribute this resource and to empower those who need it is an important goal for me. This concept, with examples, is explored more in the later part of this chapter.

Safe Places to Be Affirmed

Most academics understand that the institution has to be a place where they can boldly share ideas and have rigorous intellectual exchange in a respectful manner. But the environment may not be safe enough when there is a clash of racial realities. Difficult conversations about topics such as color blindness, meritocracy, privilege, or marginalization are challenging to navigate and may result in a clash of world-views. When such occasions arise, researchers have remarked that faculty of color find themselves in the unenviable position of processing their personal feelings while also wanting to address the emotions being expressed (Jackson, 2019; Stanley, 2006). Safe spaces allow for difficult subjects to be discussed openly without the risk of disrespect and harsh judgment. Scholars have indicated that being aware of power, racial, and ethnic assumptions and attitudes plays a vital role in creating safe spaces in which to have difficult dialogue (Chang et al., 2014). Like chipping away at a boulder, it will take many conversations with different groups, mostly well-meaning ones, to draw out the destructive nature of taken-for-granted discourses and to change perspectives.

Spiritually Connected

Social location in the spiritual sense is defined as communion with the sacred—that is, God (Pargament, 2007). For me, spirituality is associated with thoughts, feelings, and behaviors in relation to honoring and relating to the God in the Bible. "On some days … we have to know that … God has us covered because everything around us is telling us we are not really good enough" (Chang et al., 2014, p. 382). This is applicable to academia. Researchers Thomas and Hollenshead (2001) remark that female minority faculty members are more likely than are white women and men in other groups to be judged harshly for any sign of failure by their colleagues. Further, these faculty leaders are likely to be penalized more for any mistakes; these mistakes may be misconstrued as lack of capability or as intellectual inferiority.

I certainly felt this way sometimes—as if colleagues were waiting to catch my mistakes. It was present not only in my academic work, but also in others' evaluations of me. I have practiced clinically in my field's industry for many years. I took on a full teaching load and still published in several top journals. I initiated several symposia at national conferences and served on regional and national boards. I managed the mental health graduate programs. Yet, there were many occasions when someone said or did something that made me feel like a second-class citizen. For instance, despite my achievements and my role in the programs I oversaw, I was reduced to a generic word—"ladies"—in emails sent to all the administrative assistants. As another example, some student-related decisions passed me by when my approval should have been sought.

As a female leader of color, it was important that I be viewed and respected as a leader who has succeeded based on merit, but instead I sometimes found myself discounted because of my gender, race, and ethnicity. Those were the "some days" when I would let go and let God. This spiritual connection was necessary for me to continue making progress in my professional and personal development despite tiring circumstances. God knew how to handle what I could not.

Bridging the Divide

It is important that faculty of color are trying to negotiate their different identities and build more inclusive networks (Moore, 2017). Building a community of practice among faculty leaders of color is a good thing. As individuals in the group interact and communicate, they can further develop this professional community, and ultimately mentor and guide the next generation. Diversity among a group of professionals offers a realistic microcosm of the world we live in and the possibility of a different vision. It encompasses multiparty negotiation to work together to achieve a collective goal. However, diversity slows the process down, particularly when we are attempting to mix race, gender, immigration status, and class in community. There is no way to have diverse people in a room and not have people make mistakes. In fact, there will be enormous room for misunderstanding. Even with the best of intentions, all can stumble. As someone once said, "There is no dishonor in being wrong and learning. There is dishonor in willful ignorance and there is dishonor in disrespect."

Bringing groups together based on complex, intersecting identities requires commitment and competency. Research suggests that faculty leaders of color support people of all backgrounds by being positive role models, bringing to the institution the societal reality of diversity, and reflecting the interest of the institution in people of color (Hassouneh & Thomas, 2018). At every institution where I worked, I engaged with both faculty and students (of color and White) in presentations, writing projects, and conversations at many conferences. Moving forward with others from diverse backgrounds has helped me understand how, in spite of the seemingly endless stream of negativity surrounding it, the journey of inclusion and generativity will bear its reward. I see this type of engagement as part of social responsibility I owe to the many marginalized groups that have claimed me in their membership. It makes my heart joyful to engage people in this process.

Being Generative

For me, experiences based on the intersections of social locations and professional roles have been valuable and impactful. They have taught me lessons that I want to pass on to the people after me—my students, fellow junior colleagues, and the professional community. It is my way to change the trajectory of others for the better.

Participation in these opportunities has allowed me to pick up the baton of mentoring for other people of color in academia. For instance, I was there for a newer colleague of color who was disappointed and hurting because of negative student evaluations. I have been in a similar predicament and completely understood where he was coming from. This was also a reflection of insufficient training for faculty in higher education. Despite his efforts to address issues in class, a few students requested that he not teach their courses in the future. Utterly depressed and paralyzed by those evaluations, he still made a choice to improve. I took those matters seriously. I investigated to give students a fair hearing, and I decided to mentor and support the male colleague for both his own good and the students' sake.

The importance of gender, race, and ethnicity has strengthened my commitment to being a faculty leader who stimulates conversation about these issues. This means acknowledging the diverse identities that exist within our communities and recognizing power and disadvantages as systemically situated in the worlds of our graduate students. Training students to closely examine the intersectionality of social locations ignites their curiosity about how to do work that is inclusive of multiple voices and how to create new meanings and lived experiences. This includes valuing cultural knowledge from traditionally marginalized communities, as well as emphasizing the significance of drawing on knowledge informed by other home cultures, regions, and migrant experiences to enhance the professional growth of students who are marginalized. Empirical studies by professionals of color suggest that those in higher positions could consider using their acquired power to alleviate the complex oppressions experienced by different individuals (Chase, 1995; Turner, 2002). Further, upwardly mobile professionals of color frequently express a sense of responsibility to use acquired power for the good of the group (Chase, 1995). In my position of power, it is imperative to do something about the discrimination experienced by students who are marginalized.

Occupying a position that allows me to do something about others' experiences of inequality has made me more intentional about creating safe spaces to share personal stories as well as conversations about social justice and identity exploration (Sue et al., 2011). In my earlier years in higher education, I did this by inviting faculty of color from different institutions to join me in sharing their stories at national conferences organized by the American Family Therapy Association, National Council of Family Relations, etc. This type of platform allows individuals to voice what they think and begin to practice some new ways of coping. A few years ago, I shifted, continuing to build team symposia, but now with the inclusion of White colleagues. Through my work within and outside the university setting, I hope I am modeling leadership from the place of my social location in a manner that is consistent in focus and that clearly conveys my passion for creating meaningful growth environments for all.

What Have I Become?

The journey continues. My experiences as an educator, clinical director, researcher, and program director well prepare me to work with multiple levels of hierarchy, some better and others less so, to consult and develop in the field I am passionate about. My lived experience gives me open-mindedness and a new awareness of how social location in all its complexity influences my professional journey. I am committed to fostering meaningful relationships with colleagues both within and outside my institution. I also need to be myself with my colleagues. This courageous narrative helps me break down barriers for others who might be in the same boat. Yes, my gender, racial, ethnic, and immigration identities come with certain stereotypes, and I am aware it might be energy-draining. But I have a responsibility to interrupt imbalanced systemic and relational dynamics whenever I can. Particularly by leveraging my privileged position as an educated and currently able-bodied cis-female with a Christian background, I have learned to raise my voice to systems that might disproportionately impact others.

Acknowledgment I thank Dr. Carmen Knudson-Martin who took me under her wings when I first started my academic journey—opening my eyes to new stages of opportunity to grow in my scholarship, showing me how to stand my ground and have the kind of career that I can be proud of, and modeling for me how to mentor. Also I am grateful to the Fantastic Five—a name we gave to ourselves when we came together as Asian American professors learning how to negotiate and navigate uncharted waters amidst the multiple complex social locations. So thank you, Dr. Sherry Shi-Ruei Fang, Dr. Xiaolin Xie, Dr. SeongEun Kim, and Dr. Yan Ruth Xia.

References

Alexander, R., Jr., & Moore, E. S. (2008). Introduction to African Americans: Benefits and challenges of working at predominantly white institutions: Strategies for thriving. *Journal of African American Studies, 12*(1), 1.

Chase. (1995). *Ambiguous empowerment: The work narratives of women school superintendents.* Amherst, MA: University of Massachusetts Press.

Chang, H., Longman, K. A., & Franco, M. A. (2014). Leadership development through mentoring in higher education: A collaborative autoethnography of leaders of color. *Mentoring & Tutoring: Partnership in Learning, 22*(4), 373–389.

Eby, L. T., & Allen, T. D. (2008). Moving toward interdisciplinary dialogue in mentoring scholarship: An introduction to the special issue. *Journal of Vocational Behavior, 72*(2), 159–167.

Griffin, K. A., & Reddick, R. J. (2011). Surveillance and sacrifice: Gender differences in the mentoring patterns of Black professors at predominantly White research universities. *American Educational Research Journal, 48*(5), 1032–1057. https://doi.org/10.3102/0002831211405025.

Hardy, K. V. (2018). The self of the therapist in epistemological context: A multicultural relational perspective. *Journal of Family Psychotherapy, 29*(1), 17–29. https://doi.org/10.1080/0897535 3.2018.1416211.

Harris, J. R. A., Trepal, H., Prado, A., & Robinson, J. (2019). Women counselor educators' experiences of microaggressions. *Journal of Counselor Preparation & Supervision, 12*(2), 189–215.

Hassouneh, D., & Thomas, C. R. (2018). *Faculty of color in the health professions: Stories of survival and success.* Hanover, NH: Dartmouth College Press.

Jackson, J. M. (2019). Breaking out of the ivory tower: (Re)thinking inclusion of women and scholars of color in the academy. *Journal of Women, Politics & Policy, 40*(1), 195–203.

Lumby, J., & Coleman, M. (2007). *Leadership and diversity: Challenging theory and practice in education.* Thousand Oaks, CA: Sage Publications.

Moore, M. R. (2017). Women of color in the academy: Navigating multiple intersections and multiple hierarchies. *Social Problems, 64*(2), 200–205.

Morin, A., Duhnych, C., & Racy, F. (May 2018). Self-reported inner speech use in university students. *Applied Cognitive Psychology, 32*(3), 376–382. https://doi.org/10.1002/acp.3404.

Nash, J. C. (2008). Rethinking intersectionality. *Feminist Review, 89,* 1–15.

Pargament, K. I. (2007). *Spiritually integrated psychotherapy: Understanding and addressing the sacred.* New York, NY: Guilford Press.

Phillips, K. W., Rothbard, N. P., & Dumas, T. L. (2009). To disclose or not to disclose? Status distance and self-disclosure in diverse environments. *Academy of Management Review, 34*(4), 710–732.

Ponjuan, L., Conley, V. M., & Trower, C. (2011). Career stage differences in pre-tenure track faculty perceptions of professional and personal relationships with colleagues. *The Journal of Higher Education, 82,* 319–346.

Raukko, T. (2020). *Asian American Outlook. A matter of survival: Navigating media during the COVID-19 pandemic.* Intertrend. https://medium.com/intertrend/asian-american-outlook-a-matter-of-survival-navigating-media-during-the-covid-19-pandemic-c6497e41a9f.

Stanley, C. A. (2006). Coloring the academic landscape. *American Educational Research Journal, 43,* 701–736.

Sue, D. W., Rivera, D. P., Watkins, N. L., Kim, R. H., Kim, S., & Williams, C. D. (2011). Racial dialogues: Challenges faculty of color face in the classroom. *Cultural Diversity and Ethnic Minority Psychology, 17*(3), 331–340.

Thomas, G. D., & Hollenshead, C. (2001). Resisting from the margins: The coping strategies of Black women and other women of color faculty members at a research university. *Journal of Negro Education, 70*(3), 166–175. https://doi.org/10.2307/3211208.

Turner, C. (2002). Women of color in academe: Living with multiple marginality. *The Journal of Higher Education, 73*(1), 74–93.

Wong, F., & Halgin, R. (2006). The "Model Minority": Bane or blessing for Asian Americans? *Journal of Multicultural Counseling and Development, 34,* 38–49.

Chapter 3
A Rare Professor: Processing Social Location as a Taiwanese American Male in Academia and Clinical Training

Alexander Lin Hsieh

With feelings of relief, accomplishment, and some exhaustion, I look upon the audience of smiling faces; some words of appreciation, some audience members applauding, and others with inquisitive looks probably momentarily coming to the podium with questions or comments. I have just completed another workshop presentation on cultural humility, a topic I have presented on since the beginning of my academic career. While I know I will present on topics of diversity, multiculturalism, and its subtexts again, I cannot help but think whether this topic picked me or I actively decided to present on such a safe topic. Cultural diversity, multiculturalism, and cultural humility are current and discussion worthy topics in the field of Marriage and Family Therapy. It often brings heated discussion for political correctness and demonstrates our mental health value for inclusivity and equity. As I connect with supportive and enthusiastic colleagues at this national conference, I can't help but feel torn between my passions for this topic of discussion and wonder if being Taiwanese American both privileges me to this research but also limits me to it.

Throughout the history of Asian Americans, there have been many themes of Asian American men being emasculated from a social context perspective (Chan, 1991; Takaki, 1998). The cultural perspective associated with Asian American manliness has been associated with only achievement and financial success. Although mental health professionals have advocated for concepts such as empathy, vulnerability, and emotional connection, little literature focuses on these concepts with Asian American men. Furthermore, one would be hard-pressed to find literature on how to navigate the field of MFT as an Asian American male therapist, partly because Asian American men represent one of the lowest percentages of therapists today (Data USA, 2017). While several publications have focused on working with Asian American individuals (Leong & Kalibatseva, 2011; Shibusawa & Chung,

A. L. Hsieh (✉)
Couple and Family Therapy Program, Alliant International University, Sacramento, CA, USA
e-mail: ahsieh@alliant.edu

© Springer Nature Switzerland AG 2021
K. M.-T. Quek, A. L. Hsieh (eds.), *Intersectionality in Family Therapy Leadership*, AFTA SpringerBriefs in Family Therapy,
https://doi.org/10.1007/978-3-030-67977-4_3

2009; Wang & Kim, 2010) and families (Atwood & Conway, 2004; Lim & Nakamoto, 2008; Pandya & Herlihy, 2009), few researchers have concentrated on Asian American men therapist development. Quek and Chen's (2017) qualitative study looked at Chinese therapists (including five males) in training, but from the context of China rather than Western culture. In this chapter, I perceive my role in academia as a program and clinical director for Alliant International University's Couple and Family Therapy program through the lens of intersectionality (Case, Iuzzini, & Hopkins, 2012; Chenfeng, Kim, Wu, & K-M, 2017) between my Taiwanese American culture, gender identity, and social location. The social location under examination consists of structural power stemming from my academic position and of my residential geographic location of Sacramento, California. Through this perspective, I hope to convey an understanding of social location and delineate how I navigate my function and role in academia as a Taiwanese American man.

Emigration Toward Achievement

My mother emigrated to the USA from Taiwan in the late 1970s and then met and married my father in Hawaii. There they started a family and soon moved to Texas for more opportunities. I grew up in a suburban area of Dallas, Texas, with some diversity but like most suburbs of Dallas at the time, dominated by White culture. Contrary to what many thought of our family at the time, we did not have "family jewels that we carried over from China." Wealth was not something my family had. Instead, welfare, food stamps, and public transportation were commonplace in my early childhood. My mother valiantly tried her best to shield me and my sister from the feelings of living without. Actually, it was not until much later that I realized in fact we were rather poor. As early as I could remember, my mother showed us the concept of hard work, frugality, and most importantly, doing well in school. Eventually, my family worked into a middle-class income family and much later even into upper middle-class. Although our family did not have a specific religious or spiritual value, many of our Taiwanese values mirrored more Buddhist teachings: wisdom, kindness, patience, generosity, and compassion (Kibra, 2002). Above all, the value of education reigns supreme, as the main purpose for my mom's original immigration was to provide her future children a better opportunity for education.

The question "What do you want to be when you grow up?" always circulates in my mind whenever I reflect upon my career in academia as a professor, clinical director, and program director for an MFT program. For most of my childhood and early adulthood life, the answer to that question was consistently "a medical doctor, of course." More specifically, it was a cardiothoracic surgeon. The idea was one passed down and drilled in by my mother. Back in her time and into the early 2000s, Taiwan had a very challenging college application process. While many high school students desired to enter the prestigious Taiwan universities, high achieving students saturated entrance exams, coupled with limited prestigious university admissions, lead to a low percentage of success. The United States had a much different process which gave more opportunities. That was my family's American dream: the opportunity to enter a prestigious college, to seek a medical degree, and to establish a legacy on family, success, and generosity. While many Asian American families saw the big four occupations—medical doctor, engineer, lawyer, and pharmacist (Takaki, 1998)—as the only acceptable college degrees, my mom limited us to just a medical doctor. My parental expectations were very narrow, and ultimately, my career choice deviated heavily from cultural and familial expectations. Not only did my career choice not fall within cultural expectations, but the decision also deviated from normal cultural patterns of filial piety. Ironically, my decision to pursue a career in marriage and family therapy was supplanted by Taiwanese values; the belief that the family system mattered and was worth talking about. I gravitated toward MFT because of how important I see relationshipss and how much we can achieve through healthy relationships.

Unfortunately, navigating through this field as a Taiwanese American man lacked role models and contained many foreign concepts, such as differentiation, the family circumplex model, and self-care, which are unique to Western cultures, but contradicted Asian values such as: collectivism, family enmeshment, and being self-sacrificing (Hynes, 2019). The esteemed Insoo Berg Kim was one of few major role models who confirmed the possibility that Asian Americans can contribute to a mostly Westernized social science. Understanding my family's emigration story paves my perspective on my identity as a clinical director and program director. As I conceptualize my social location, I will be speaking on two fronts: the microlevel perspective within Sacramento (a Northern California diverse urban community) and the macrolevel of a Taiwanese American male in the field of marriage and family therapy education. Both the micro and macrolevel assessment contributes to my continuous internal dialogue.

My Social Location

For this chapter, I will be addressing social location in accordance to two administrative roles I hold in my profession. The context of these roles will be evaluated based on my current residence of Sacramento, but I must also acknowledge that my social location has changed, given my pursuit in my academic career as I will discuss later. My role as program director for an MFT program reveals areas of privilege and systemic power that I must navigate throughout my role with students. As my program's clinical director, I must also be mindful of how my cultural values, expectations, and identity interact with my work with the local Sacramento community, a diverse population with mental health access and funding difficulties. At the microlevel, my social location revolves around the physical setting of Sacramento, California, one of the most diverse cities in the United States, capital to one of the most influential states with a high concentration of MFTs, and a city that, like many, struggles to find value in mental health, which is reflected in limited grant funding and political support. On the macrolevel, I consider the values of the MFT field and context of MFT training. I utilize an intersectional model (Chenfeng et al., 2017; Mahalingam, 2007) lens specific to my identity as a Taiwanese American man interacting with my social location and perceive how they influence my academia position and internal processing.

The Asian American Cultural Bubble

Often times, the Asian American community talks about the Asian American bubble both in positive and negative ways. Let me start by saying that, to me, the Asian American bubble comes from a place of privilege because in my life, it mostly has been a social choice to stay in the bubble rather than one which is forced like gentrification. The Asian American bubble may start with social interactions early in teenage and young adult years and be perpetuated by one's family involvement within the Asian American community, and then grows into social and residential segregation in adulthood. In my early teenage and college years, I was in the Asian American bubble. I socialized exclusively with Asian Americans (mostly Chinese, Taiwanese, Korean, and Japanese Americans), only had Asian American roommates, predominately ate Asian cuisine, studied with an all-Asian American study group, and often times only had to speak Mandarin, if I chose to. When non-Asian individuals entered our social bubble, it was looked upon with suspicion and concern. Looking back, it was not a proud moment for me, but it did breed levels of comfort, safety, and a strong sense of belonging; all things I was searching for early on. This concept has become more difficult for me to grasp now because of my strong belief in promoting diversity, multiculturalism, and inclusivity to facilitate difficult dialogues and improve mental health throughout our communities. Change happened as I got older and experienced ever-changing social locations.

Even as I began my MFT education, there was a social bubble I meant to impact. I wanted to pursue a career in MFT to connect with Asian American individuals, couples, and families. I wanted to break down why Asian Americans were the least likely to utilize mental health services (Kim, 2007; Kim, Ng, & Ahn, 2005; US Department of Health and Human Services, 2001), end the stigma in Asian culture that seeking mental health services is a sign of weakness, and help Asian couples find higher levels of marital satisfaction. The course of my education took me to two predominantly White homogeneous cities (Abilene, Texas and Provo, Utah) largely absent of the Asian American bubble. At first, I was very resistant to change, and it brought me little joy. Finally, my academic position placed me in one of the most diverse cities in the nation. At that point, I had to make a difficult decision for myself: either reestablish the Asian American bubble or utilize the diverse location and not only make an impact in Asian American mental health, but an impact to promote diversity within mental health and decrease stigma of mental health across race and ethnicities.

Although it may seem like an easy decision to make, it was difficult for me because for the first time, my position of power as a faculty member with PhD status allowed for more action and change to occur, and that seemed terrifying in a community I was not accustomed to. In addition, it somehow felt like a betrayal to my Asian American community. It was not comfortable. One occurrence especially comes to mind—when I entered a Black community panel discussion involving social injustice, police brutality, and how mental health agencies can be more effective with the black community. I was an outsider going into a community that has been suffering and hurting. The community was angry, frustrated, outraged, and wanted change. When I was first introduced, I perceived a deep sense of judgment and disconnection from that community. Although my first instinct was to build credibility with my research, accolades, university position, and education level, a part of me knew that would create more disconnection and potentially even disdain. So, I took a page out of the Sue and Sue's (2016) research I so held dearly and asked for the opportunity to listen to the community. I listened, and listened, and continued to listen as individuals and families talked about the generations and multiple instances of how the various mental health systems have failed them. My panelist role inverted to being a member of the audience, and I loved it!

Throughout the discussion, I had to follow multicultural practice (Sue & Sue, 2016) and check my privilege repeatedly. My Taiwanese culture wanted to say "you see the problem, don't just complain about it, pull yourself up by your bootstraps and do something about it. Better yourself, and if you can't, that is your own fault." As more stories were shared, I began to resent this part of me more. How could a part of me lack so much empathy? I quickly differentiated that this part of me has always been present, and it was an important part of who I am and how I got to where I am today. Although I would never say my academic position is something to brag about (Taiwanese humility), it was a goal I had, and obtaining my academic position was an achievement. Internally, I had to process and check this privileged part of me, stemming from my cultural upbringing, at the door when I came back for round two of a similar discussion. Only through this struggle and first seeing my privilege could I better empathize with my community and begin working with the community's many struggles, which I may not be directly impacted by but frequently am a part of based on my geographic location alone.

This experience marked a tremendous epiphany for me because for the first time, I was able to step out of my created Asian American bubble and see my privilege and use that privilege to work with a marginalized community in desperate need of mental health reform. I would not say we made tremendous changes, but I believe the discussions were rich and fueled community action to build connections around mental health and the Black community. I believe that, although my cultural bubble bred safety, comfort, and familiarity, my education and training begged me to participate with my community rather than continue to seclude. As I articulate this belief, I realize even that choice was one of privilege. My social location coupled with the privilege of my educational training propelled me to learn and do better.

It is with this perspective that I keep engaging with my community and my role as a clinical director. This role serves as a connection between the mental health agencies, communities accessing mental health services, my university, and our program's students. It is within my job description to develop community agency sites where our students can gain clinical practicum experience. I believe this is a pivotal role in any MFT program because students' first experience as an MFT therapist relies on the populations that their community mental health agencies serve. That experience can vary from more homogeneous client populations like a private practice from a high-SES community setting to a very diverse population such as a transitional homeless community shelter.

My role as a clinical director bestows a great deal of power. What I choose with that power may dictate accessibility of mental health services albeit on a small scale. My experience interacting with my community has taught me that although my students may not always feel the most comfortable in gaining experience in these communities of need, it is certainly my obligatory duty bestowed by my social location to connect my students, my program, and at times supervision, research, and consultation to mental health agencies focused on serving marginalized populations. Just like that, my Asian American cultural bubble not only burst, but from it paved way for a new and more inclusive bubble. Fortunately, this new bubble resonated more with my newly learned core beliefs and resonates better with MFT's core values.

My Three Ps: Problems, Power, and Privilege

It would be an oversight to discuss social location without examining power and privilege. Ironically, I have considered many Asian American stereotypes from a perspective of privilege. The major one being the model minority concept originating from William Peterson, a sociologist who writes for *The New York Times Magazine* in the mid-1960s (Chan, 1991; Takaki, 1998). What followed was a series of success stories published by various newspapers and magazines, detailing the various challenges, persistence, and achievement of predominantly Asian Americans. The concept is now associated with high socioeconomic success, lower rates of criminality, and high familial stability. The dark side of the model minority stereotype alludes to suggestions that as a whole, the Asian American population should not receive governmental assistance or programs, and further breeds divide between minority groups. In addition, individual Asian Americans who do not achieve to the expectations of the model minority status tend to be ostracized. While those constant expectations and achievement levels have plagued my adolescent and young adult life, my social location perspective has provided some levels of privilege.

The model minority stereotypes cast the shadow of family and marital stability upon me. Although also a stereotype, being a marriage and family therapist clinician, teaching for an MFT program and obtaining my PhD in Marriage and Family Therapy already projects such traits. It is natural, albeit flawed, to believe that such an individual would have family and marital stability; just like it would be to expect a medical doctor to always have good healthy habits, a personal trainer to be in immaculate physical shape, or a pastor to be spiritually grounded. Based on this stereotype, I believe it has granted me a privilege because of the alignment between MFT's focus on family systems and the model minority assumptions.

It has felt that I have found my place in my community of mental health focused on generating healthy, stable, safety, and secure relationships between partners and family members. It becomes easy and almost natural to advocate for my students to conduct family therapy and couple therapy because of this stereotype. Often when I am creating agency partnerships for students' practicum, systemic therapy is not always a method agencies are familiar with or can necessarily implement. Many past MFT researchers have found support that systemic therapy is actually effective and often more cost-effective than individualized treatment (Crane & Christenson, 2014; Goorden et al., 2016), but agencies still sometimes need convincing. I believe this is one area which my model minority privilege, based on the stereotypes of achievement, success, and strong family values, opens the conversation with part-nered agencies to allow my students to conduct systemic family therapy. This trend tends to happen effortlessly, which I credit to the intersection of the model minority stereotypes and my credential as an MFT professor. Considering how mental health funding seem to be decreasing year after year, especially in a city like Sacramento, where advocacy and lobbying for other issues are just as rampant, consistently find-ing a place for systemic therapy in the community is not guaranteed, but a focus on therapeutic achievement and success seems to resonate with many community men-tal health agencies. This privilege has given our program an abundance of practicum partnerships, essential for student training success.

What about the problems of the "model minority" stereotype? Here, I would like to take a look at the interaction between Taiwanese American culture as the model minority and culture of academia. Specifically, I want to highlight the academic culture of working endless hours producing research, improving program success data (i.e., graduation rates, student attrition, student job placement rate, etc.), and impacting your community. The interaction between these two cultural traits breeds opportunity to overwork endlessly and tirelessly.

The Unsuspecting MFT Program Director

The percentage of Asians as marriage and family therapists has and still lags far behind White Americans, Hispanic/Latino Americans, and Black/African Americans (Data USA, 2017). Within the Asian American group, males are even less repre-sented as MFTs compared to females. It is relatively rare to see an Asian American male therapist, and even rarer to have one part of an MFT program. Asian Americans have the tendency and stereotype to not express vulnerable emotions (Chan, 1991; Takaki, 1998), something that is frequently discussed in the field of psychotherapy, but absolutely crucial as a marriage and family therapist.

I remember a distinct moment in my early childhood. I must have been maybe 10 or 11 years of age. I was in Taiwan on summer vacation, where my sister and I frequently went to stay with my aunt and grandmother. I can't quite remember what I did, but I was being strongly scolded by one of my uncles. I do remember that I then began to cry, which quickly spurred my uncle to raise his voice and say in Mandarin "不能哭，男子漢 大丈夫眼淚比血更珍貴" (stop crying, a man's tears are more precious than blood). From that moment, I learned to not show emotions, hold my vulnerabilities close to my heart, and not let others see it. Of course, I now recognize that this perspective is erroneous and potentially destructive because it minimizes the importance of emotions and how emotions are a basic part of human interactions and mental health. Nearly every MFT theory emphasizes the importance of emotions, needing to recognize and validate emotions, and being able to effectively express them. It took many years, some therapy, countless hours of self-reflection, and journey through both a Master's and PhD marriage and family therapy program to overcome this aspect of my Taiwanese male stereotype.

Naturally, it would have been difficult to hold onto this stereotype and teach in an MFT program that preaches empathy, vulnerability, talking about emotions, and compassion. It would be nearly impossible, and highly hypocritical, if I held onto my uncle's words and taught or modeled entirely different therapeutic concepts to my students. As a program director, often I meet with students who are struggling with the curriculum, clinical practice, or program in general. Often times, their struggles are not because of the lack of comprehension but rather life's circumstances (i.e., working two jobs and not having time to complete homework assignments, grieving loss, natural disasters, or mental health struggles). Internally, I recognize that throughout my life, I have had to push aside disappointment, shame, heartbreak, and rejection to focus on a job, assignment, exam, or responsibilities. It never entered my mind to ever ask an employer, professor, or supervisor for accommodations because of life's circumstances. Doing so would only bring upon more shame (Hampton & Sharp, 2014) and be a sign of weakness.

In my journey in academia, many of my mentors showed me compassion and empathy rather than shaming my lack of achievement whenever I fell short. Through this model, it has propelled me to want to achieve more and not disappoint them. I believe this resonates with a more strength-based model which is prevalent in our field (Nichols & Davis, 2015). As a program director, I have to demonstrate empathy and compassion to my students, understanding that it takes more courage to talk with an authority figure and express struggles and vulnerability. While my uncle responded to my vulnerability with anger and discipline, I chose to take a different path: one of empathy and encouragement.

This foundation lends an opportunity to build a stronger connection with students and opens the door toward support and conversation, where intimidation and fear may have previously resided. Of course, I have to validate my part that does still value achievement and task completion by following up with students with "how can I support you to encourage your best work moving forward?" or "what can we do to get your best work?" I believe this method resonates with the MFT systemic model because it places a student's success in our program not squarely on the student's shoulders, but allows the burden to be supported by the program as well. This systemic perspective to promote student success also resonates with Asian collectivistic principles (Takaki, 1998). Specifically, when there is collective responsibility and cooperation to bring about student success, it also leads to program success. This deviates from individualistic perspectives, which may put the responsibility solely on the student to achieve, which strongly deviates from systems thinking, the foundation of any MFT program. There must be shared responsibilities toward the path of student training successful as a prosperous marriage and family therapist. Balance has been a strong cultural identity I have taken from my Taiwanese American heritage and incorporated into all aspects of my career in academia.

Topic of Balance

As the late Pat Morita said while playing the role of Mr. Miyagi "The lesson is not just for karate only. The lesson is for the whole life. If your whole life has balance, everything will be better." Culturally, balance is at the key center of Confucianism and Taoism, and very much rooted in Taiwanese culture (Chan, 1991; Takaki, 1998). The concept of Yin and Yang applies to all aspect of life, including health, nature, and character. Only when there is balance, does one gain the most clear perspective and is able to maximize achievement. Although I do not identify with the religious label of Buddhism, the cultural principle of balance has centered my perspective in my academic position. In addition, balance interacts with my cultural identity on achievement.

What is the balance between the rigors of my academic position and my social location? In many ways, the balance is grounded in how I can maximize and be most efficient in the work that I do. The outcome matters. Maybe that is a Taiwanese cultural bias, but success is extremely important to my identity and perception of my academic role. I also definitely understand that success for my MFT program, the students, and my mental health professional community takes a great deal of balance. The drive to push these three levels toward success is grounded in my cultural identity. As a result, I think my social location provides the perfect opportunity to achieve this success. As a program director, it allows me to make influential decisions that directly impact the success of our program and students. My role as a clinical director not only carries a responsibility for my students' success, but also the continued growth and visibility of MFT mental health. Being at the capital of California gives me opportunity for great visibility on state policies in a state, which the rest of the country often looks for leadership in mental health policies.

But what happens when we lose balance and disruptions occur? Often this can happen when social injustice reigns. I perceive this on both the internal and external fronts. Internally, what am I doing to counter these social problems? Externally, what change is happening to promote social justice? This all becomes central issues that from my position of power I feel the need to address. I am fortunate enough to be employed by an institution that values inclusivity. Specifically, my university is "committed to inclusive, excellence; [they] value, include and engage the rich diversity of the [university's] community." This synergy between my values and my university's values allows for opportunity for action to be taken to seek internal balance in hopes of external change leading to more balance.

The actions I have taken from a position of power as an MFT program director and clinical director include: supporting disadvantaged students, working with and empowering marginalized communities, and advocating for social justice. These actions bring me internal balance because social justice work is being done. The external balance is perceived when students from historically marginalized communities graduate and then inspires and gives back to their underserved communities, and also, when advocacy for social justice contributes to appropriate policy changes. Balance in my academic role is then achieved by being allowed and encouraged to incorporate topics of social justice, diversity, inclusion, and multiculturalism into program curriculum, practicum site development, course content, and program-community engagement. Our program engages and promotes collaboration with community mental health agencies centered on inclusivity. Finally, within the university, a culture of difficult dialogues, social justice and diversity education, and multicultural practice are a commonplace occurrence. This results in moments of my internal harmony even while external factors may be chaotic, disruptive, and experiencing social unrest. The balance becomes the final string that ties my Taiwanese American male identity and my social location together.

Conclusion

My journey is not done, nor do I want it to be. In my ever-changing social location, it would be extremely remise if I found comfort in where I reside today and impede my growth. When power is bestowed based on aspects of social location, leaders of our community get the opportunity to decide how that privilege is utilized. I hope that I will continue to grow and challenge my comfort level. I hope that I continue to better understand my position of privilege and use that privilege to both support and advance marginalized communities. The interaction between my cultural and gender values, my academic roles, and place of residency brings about a unique social location that can in turn change the landscape of mental health, bit by bit.

As I sit at the airport after giving my last talk on cultural humility, I recall answering questions, exchanging contact information, and discussing potential future collaboration and connections. I now sit here pondering how social location has shaped not only who I am in academia, but how I conduct myself from an administrative perspective and represent both my program and students. Fortunately, I feel empowered and privileged that my social location also allows me to affect my community both on a micro and macrolevel. So, as I board my flight home, I reflect on a sense of optimism, challenge, and career goals of bringing these experiences and knowledge gained to the MFT field and my current and future students. This purpose shall never tire me.

Acknowledgment I have to start by thanking God for blessing me with the many opportunities in my career. I want to acknowledge my loving wife, Lindsay, without her encouragement and support none of this would be possible. I also want to acknowledge my mother and sister who always push me to be my absolute best. Thanks also to all the many mentors along my academic journey who have challenged me and pushed me out of my comfort zone. Finally, thanks to all my supportive faculty and colleagues at my university who always offer tremendous support and collegiality.

References

Atwood, J. D., & Conway, B. Y. M. (2004). Therapy with Chinese American families: A social constructionist perspective. *The American Journal of Family Therapy, 32*, 155–172.

Case, K. A., Iuzzini, J., & Hopkins, M. (2012). Systems of privilege: Intersections, awareness, and applications. *Journal of Social Issues, 68*, 1–10.

Chan, S. (1991). *Asian Americans: An interpretive history*. New York, NY: Twayne Publishers.

Chenfeng, J., Kim, L., Wu, Y., & K-M, C. (2017). Addressing culture, gender, and power with Asian American couples: Application of socio-emotional relationship therapy. *Family Process, 56*(3), 558–573.

Crane, D. R., & Christenson, J. (2014). A summary report of cost-effectiveness: Recognizing the value of family therapy in healthcare. In J. Hodgson, A. Lamson, T. Mendenhall, & D. R. Crane (Eds.), *Medical family therapy: Advanced applications* (pp. 419–436). Cham, Switzerland: Springer International Publishing.

Data USA. (2017). *Marriage & family therapy*. https://datausa.io/profile/cip/marriage-family-therapy#employment.

Goorden, M., Schawo, S. J., Bouwmans-Frijters, C. A. M., van der Schee, E., Hendriks, V. M., & Roijen, L. H. (2016). The cost-effectiveness of family/family-based therapy for treatment of externalizing disorders, substance use disorders and delinquency: A systematic review. *BMS Psychiatry, 16*, 237.

Hampton, N. Z., & Sharp, S. E. (2014). Shame-focused attitudes toward mental health problems: The role of gender and culture. *Rehabilitation Counseling Bulletin, 57*(3), 170–181.

Hynes, K. C. (2019). Cultural values matter: The therapeutic alliance and East Asian Americans. *Contemporary Family Therapy, 41*, 392–400.

Kibra, N. (2002). *Becoming Asian American: Second-generation Chinese and Korean American identities*. Baltimore: The John Hopkins University Press.

Kim, B. S. K. (2007). Adherence to Asian and European American cultural values and attitudes toward seeking professional psychological help among Asian American college students. *Journal of Counseling Psychology, 54*, 474–480.

Kim, B. S. K., Ng, G. F., & Ahn, A. J. (2005). Effects of client expectation for counseling success, client-counselor worldview match, and client adherence to Asian and European American cultural values on counseling process with Asian Americans. *Journal of Counseling Psychology, 52*, 67–76.

Leong, F. T. L., & Kalibatseva, Z. (2011). Effective psychotherapy for Asian Americas: From cultural accommodation to cultural congruence. *Clinical Psychology: Science and Practice, 18*, 242–245.

Lim, S.-L., & Nakamoto, T. (2008). Genograms: Use in therapy with Asian families with diverse cultural heritages. *Contemporary Family Therapy, 30*, 199–219.

Mahalingam, R. (2007). Essentialism and cultural narratives: A social-marginality perspective. In A. J. Fuligni (Ed.), *Contesting stereotypes and creating identities: Social categories, social identities, and educational participation* (pp. 42–65). New York, NY: Russell Sage Foundation.

Nichols, M. P., & Davis, S. D. (2015). *Family therapy: Concepts and methods* (11th ed.). Upper Saddle River, NJ: Pearson Education.

Pandya, K., & Herlihy, J. (2009). An exploratory study into how a sample of a British South Asian population perceive the therapeutic alliance in family therapy. *The Association for Family Therapy and Systemic Practice, 31*, 384–404.

Quek, K. M.-T., & Chen, H.-M. (2017). Family therapy in Chinese culture and context: Lessons from supervising therapists-in-training in China. *Contemporary Family Therapy, 39*, 12–20.

Shibusawa, T., & Chung, I. W. (2009). Wrapping and unwrapping emotions: Clinical practice with East Asian immigrant elders. *Clinical Social Work Journal, 37*, 312–319.

Sue, D. W., & Sue, D. (2016). *Counseling the culturally diverse: Theory and practice*. Hoboken, NJ: Wiley.

Takaki, R. (1998). *Strangers from a different shore: A history of Asian Americans*. Boston, MA: Back Bay Books.

U.S. Department of Health and Human Services. (2001). *Mental health: Culture, race, ethnicity— A supplement to mental health: A report of the surgeon general*. Rockville, MD: Author.

Wang, S., & Kim, B. S. K. (2010). Therapist multicultural competence, Asian American participants' cultural values, and counseling process. *Journal of Counseling Psychology, 57*(4), 394–401.

Chapter 4
Power on the Margins: Navigating the Program Director Role as an Asian, Queer, Immigrant Woman in Canada

Narumi Taniguchi

"Japanese, woman, middle class, first in my family to go to university, first to study abroad, non-religious, lesbian, introvert." This is the list of identifiers that I included in one of the first slides that said "About Me." I showed this slide to my hiring committee and over 50 MFT students as part of my job talk when I interviewed for the program director position at my current Canadian university. Of all identifiers, "lesbian" went in and out of the slide a few times while preparing the talk and eventually stayed in. It was because I had no idea how it would be received, and I knew I could "pass" as straight if I chose not to include it. I had been in Canada for less than 3 years at that time and did not have any firsthand knowledge about the University's culture beyond what I gathered from its website. Some years later, one of my hiring committee members asked me if I intended to "test" them by including "lesbian" in my job talk. "Yes, I did," I answered. I have gone through similar interview processes for faculty positions several times in the past, and it was the first time that I intentionally came out at the time of the interview. I was at a point in my life and career when I knew I would not want to be part of any group where I would not be respected and valued for who I am, because *who* I am has a lot to do with *how* I am as a program director.

This chapter is about my experience as an MFT program director at a Canadian university. I will recount part of my life story to provide context for my social location. My experience is intertwined with my social location, and examples will illustrate the complexity resulting from my intersectionality (Crenshaw, 1989). Although intersectionality often makes us invisible, my newly acquired power offers visibility within the institution. I will delineate some of the ways in which my professional life in North America has changed. Lastly, this chapter will discuss my relational use of power, as I am determined not to lose myself in power.

N. Taniguchi (✉)
Master of Marriage and Family Therapy Program, The University of Winnipeg,
Winnipeg, MB, Canada
e-mail: n.taniguchi@uwinnipeg.ca

© Springer Nature Switzerland AG 2021
K. M.-T. Quek, A. L. Hsieh (eds.), *Intersectionality in Family Therapy
Leadership*, AFTA SpringerBriefs in Family Therapy,
https://doi.org/10.1007/978-3-030-67977-4_4

In this chapter, I sometimes use the word queer to describe my sexual orientation, but it describes an ideology too. A queer ideology is one that seeks to challenge dominant discourses about not only sexual orientations and gender, but also other marginalized identities (Eng, Halberstam, & Muñoz, 2005). Please note that while the stories that I tell in this chapter are real, the descriptors of the people involved have been changed to protect their identities.

Who Am I?

I was born and raised in Osaka, Japan, by parents whose marriage was arranged by a matchmaker. Different from traditional Japanese families, in which father is the head of the family, followed by the firstborn son and mother, and the daughters are the lowest in the hierarchy, my parents put me, the firstborn child and the only daughter, above their two sons. My parents were running a vegetable wholesale store and had no time for their children. My brothers and I all knew that I was in charge; my brothers were told to listen to me. My mother graduated from high school in a rural town and worked in a cosmetics store before my parents got married. My father, who grew up in the city which was chaotic in the postwar era, took university classes at night while selling vegetables at a market during the day in Osaka. They both valued education but did not know much about the hypercompetitive educational system that I had to navigate.

I made my own decisions, including which schools I would apply to and take the entrance exams for. Looking back, I was always somewhat of a risk-taker, aiming for schools that required slightly higher test scores than my ability. I had the privilege of knowing that my parents would support me with whatever decisions I made. It took me two extra years to pass the entrance exam and get into the university of my dreams. I graduated from university with a B.A. in Education. My plan was to become an elementary school teacher, but instead I decided to go to graduate school in the USA because I wanted to be a family therapist. I was the first person in my entire family to not only go to graduate school, but also live outside of Japan. I went to the USA all by myself, with no relatives or friends to rely on. Because I was learning to work, write, and think in a second language, it took me 5 years, twice the normal program length, to graduate with a master's degree in Marriage and Family Therapy from a university in New York State. Those 5 years were like walking upside down, learning to do things differently, often the opposite of how I was taught: speaking up vs. "silence is golden," getting to the point vs. beating around the bush, thinking of oneself vs. thinking of others first, independent vs. interdependent, etc. During this time, I also realized for the first time in my life that I was a lesbian.

Upon graduation, I went back to Osaka and worked as a counselor in an outpatient psychiatric clinic. I was quickly promoted to assistant director of the counseling division. Experiencing reverse cultural shock, I tried to fit back into the Japanese culture and way of doing things and yet was perceived as "Americanized" by my boss at work, friends, and family. I began exploring lesbian communities in Japan and was "out" to some of my colleagues and friends. Four years later, I returned to the USA to pursue a Ph.D. degree in Texas with the goal of training MFTs in Japan.

At that time, I made a decision not to be "out" because it might have put me at risk, and getting a Ph.D. degree was more important to me than being open about my sexual orientation. It was also because being one of the few students of color would be more than enough to handle while going through the Ph.D. program in a small city in Texas. It was in the acknowledgments in my doctoral dissertation that I finally came out, quietly.

Just before completing my Ph.D., I got my first job in academia as faculty of an MFT program in California. It was a dream come true, not in Japan but in the USA. I worked there for 6 years, until I left the USA to move to Canada. I lived in the USA for a total of 18 years as a nonresident "alien" and chose to pursue permanent residency in Canada. Once again, I made the move all by myself, with no relatives or friends in Canada. I got another faculty job in an undergraduate program at a Montreal university, where I learned Québecois French culture as an allophone, hidden among Anglophones. Three years later, I was offered the current MFT program director position at a university on the Canadian Prairies. I moved halfway across the country to a midsize city that I had not known existed.

It is important to highlight additional privileges that are granted to me living in North America. As a resident alien or a permanent resident, my social location is different from other people of color in North America who have experienced colonization as groups and continue to experience various manifestations of colonialism. It should be clear in my brief life journey that I chose to move to the USA and immigrate to Canada; nobody forced me to come to North America. Moody (2011) argues the importance of distinguishing immigrants from domestic colonized groups. Certain Asian groups have privileges and are given the status of "model minority" or "honorary white" (Moody, 2011). I have experienced microaggressions and systemic oppression since I moved to North America, but they are not the same as other nonimmigrant groups experience every day for their entire lives and generationally. It is important to note here that Japanese Americans and Japanese Canadians were sent to internment camps during and after WWII, even though they were already established in their respective countries, and their lives have been impacted for generations (Hashimoto, 2012; Nagata, Kim, & Nguyen, 2015). I am not part of those groups and do not have anyone in my extended family who is impacted by the internment atrocity directly or indirectly. I do not carry any of the historic traumas that other people of color and even some Japanese Americans and Japanese Canadians carry. I have known all along that I could always go back to my country if things became unbearable. That is one of the privileges that I have as someone who chose to relocate to North America.

Where Am I?

When I first was invited to write my lived experience as an MFT program director for this book on intersectionality, identity, and power, the image of the infamous traffic junction in the city where I live called Confusion Corner came to mind. As its name implies, Confusion Corner is where several streets meet at odd angles. It is difficult for drivers who are not familiar with the area to navigate; I too have struggled to get into the correct lane and ended up on the wrong street more than once. Literature uses the term "labyrinth" to describe the complexities that women in leadership have to navigate (Ayman & Korabik, 2010; Sanchez-Hucles & Davis, 2010). In a labyrinth, there is one way in and one way out. With Confusion Corner, however, there are multiple entrances and exits, and you never know if you are on the right path until you get close to the intersection, unless you have someone famil- iar with the area guiding you. Crenshaw (1989) theorizes that "the intersectional experience is greater than the sum of racism and sexism" (p. 140). She notes that "if an accident happens in an intersection, it can be caused by cars traveling from any number of directions and, sometimes, from all of them" (p. 140). To return to the Confusion Corner metaphor, if I were to get into an accident in the intersection and be injured, my injury could be caused by patriarchy, white supremacy, homophobia, xenophobia, or all of them. The problem is that I would not know for certain which one. Sanchez-Hucles and Davis (2010) argue that it would be difficult for women of color to respond appropriately when they may not know which aspect caused the other's reaction. To make the matters worse, in my current position of power, I would be driving a bus with passengers, and a collision could cause harm to others. Below are examples to illustrate this complexity.

Every year, my program holds information sessions for people who are inter- ested in applying or want to know more about the program. I do most of the program presentation while a junior faculty member covers some parts. In one of the ses- sions, a participant, a white man, asked several questions over the course of the event. After a few questions, it became clear to me that he would look at me when asking questions and quickly turn to the junior faculty, who is a white man, for the answers. I was standing in front of the room, and my colleague was sitting to the side. I was annoyed by this participant's behavior because it was as if he was saying, "I know you're the program director, but you don't count. The male professor should know what he is talking about. I trust him more." I observed this back and forth between the two men for some time, and eventually interrupted my colleague who began to respond and instead answered the question that was asked of me. In this example, I am almost certain that the white male participant manifested misogyny, white supremacy, or both, but I cannot know which. Had I been certain that his behavior was triggered by my gender, not by my race, I would have sought some support from and/or comradery with women colleagues who are mostly white. I did not share this experience with anyone because I was afraid that my white women colleagues would make it a race issue, perhaps suggesting that my Asian "timid- ness" was the reason for the man's behavior, or attend only to the sexism aspect of what happened. My experience is that people not at the intersection of race and gender have difficulty understanding the compounding effect and choose to focus on one or the other.

I was accustomed to my invisibility. People of color often try to minimize the signs of differences and make others comfortable in white institutions (Ahmed, 2012). Coupled with this, women of color are not seen because they are doubly out of the norm in terms of gender and race (Purdie-Vaughns & Eibach, 2008). The paradox is that with the program director position, however, I often have to be "on" (Nixon, 2017). I thought I was finally visible, but this white male participant reminded me that even when holding a position of power, I can still be invisible in public while standing in front of a roomful of people, and it is a humiliating experience.

I also encounter this kind of erasure of my expertise at times when I am interacting with students who come to see me with program-related questions. Sometimes, even if I provide the clearest answer possible and students seem satisfied, I observe them going immediately to ask my white male colleague the same question. In these moments, I want to say, "What makes you think this colleague, who is not even an administrator, knows more about the program than I do?" This would be a good supervision question if I was their supervisor. However, with over 100 students in the program, I do not have the level of connection required to have such conversations with most students. Instead, I usually let it go. The risk of being perceived as controlling and/or abusing power seems too high from where I stand as program director. In these cases, I cannot tell which aspect of my identity makes students question my knowledge of the program. These experiences underscore for me that nobody can escape from the structural inequality (e.g., misogyny and white supremacy) deeply embedded in North American societies (Bishop, 2015). Everyone, regardless of their identity, can manifest racism and/or sexism unintentionally, trusting the opinion of less qualified white men than women of color because they are internalizing a lifetime of invalidating and erasing the voices of women and people of color.

The following example illustrates a similar dilemma in intersectional complexity. Two of the three major aspects of my identity, woman and Asian, are visible in North America. Although I have been mistaken for Chinese many times, people do identify me as an Asian woman. My queerness on the other hand is not as visible as I would like it to be. I can pass as straight, even when I am with my partner who is white and visibly queer. We often encounter people whose reaction to us suggests that they cannot fathom that we are a couple. In the grocery store checkout line, we are almost always asked if we want to pay separately for our cart full of groceries that we are unloading together. Heterosexuality is the norm, and those of us who are outside of the norm continue to have to constantly come out if we want to be ourselves. I suspect that the heterosexual assumption is even stronger for Asian women. During a public talk that I gave as program director, I thanked my partner for her help and support. I was aware that some people in the audience did not know my sexual orientation. After the talk, a white man who is affiliated with the university approached me and said that he too applied for the program director position. He said with excitement, "You have lots of diversity! No wonder you were selected for the position." I froze with disbelief and kept smiling. It was appalling to me that this person told me to my face that I got the program director job because of my identity, not because of my qualification, experience, knowledge, etc. He managed to reduce me to an affirmative action hire (Turner, González, & Wong 2011) in order to explain to me why he did not get my job. I contemplated the idea of having a conversation with him later. In the end, I chose not to talk with him for at least two reasons. Firstly, I thought there was a risk that he would accuse me of overreacting and would tell me that I misunderstood his comment. Secondly, I was concerned that with my relative power as program director, my intervention might be perceived as chastising rather than conversational, especially by someone who did not think he did anything wrong.

Unintentional devaluation of abilities on the basis of identity should be familiar to anyone who is on the margins of North American society. These examples highlight the effects of multiple marginality and its intersection with power afforded to me by virtue of having a middle management position at my institution.

Can You See Me?

My experience as a queer Asian woman faculty in North America can be summed up with one word: invisible. People do not remember me or my name unless I work directly with them. There were times that I felt that colleagues forgot that I even existed. Intersectional invisibility is experienced by people with multiple marginality of their identity because they are not the prototype of any groups to which they are supposed to belong (Purdie-Vaughns & Eibach, 2008). On the contrary, the program director role requires one to be visible within the institution. I was proud the first time the president of my university recognized me off campus, said my name, and asked me about the state of the program. It still surprises and delights me every time this happens.

There are two ways in which I realized that the power I now have has changed my social location. Power has always been presented as something negative, to avoid, and not to wish for throughout my life as a woman who was raised in a collectivist culture. In a study of Asian Americans in leadership positions, Kawahara, Pal, and Chin (2013) found that participants described their leadership style as "collaborative and group oriented" (p. 244). As an MFT who went through my training after the field was hit by a wave of postmodernism (Wieling et al., 2001), I was trained to be aware of the power that therapists innately have over clients and to respect clients' knowledge and experience (D'Arrigo-Patrick, Hoff, Knudson-Martin, & Tuttle, 2017). I have always been mindful of the power that I have over students as faculty; at the same time, I had to work to earn their respect by presenting some authority because of the way I know people sometimes perceive/treat women and/or Asians and/or queer people. In my current role as program director, I realized that students are actually intimidated by me, no matter how hard I try to be approachable and friendly. Several students have said that they see me as someone on a pedestal, to my surprise. I had to recognize that it takes a significant amount of courage for students to reach out to me and that I need to consider the power imbalance while also asserting authority.

One of the positive shifts that I have experienced was through various meetings with the university's senior administrators. As a faculty accustomed to being invisible, I was so used to my voice not being heard, but that changed with my current title. I inherited an MFT program that lost its COAMFTE accreditation a few years before I was hired. The program had a long history of operating as an independent

MFT training institute loosely connected to the university. My primary responsibility as program director was to get the program reaccredited, which included restructuring the program and integrating it into the university system. I was the only full-time faculty for the first 3 years, and often worked directly with senior administration to make necessary changes. I have made many suggestions and written several proposals leading to the program's major structural changes. In these meetings, I realized that I was seen and heard. I was in fact amazed every time my suggestions were taken seriously by senior administration.

The newly acquired visibility that accompanied the program director position has been empowering. I can see how people get used to the power and become power-hungry. It is also frightening to carry the enormous responsibilities of being part of decision-making units and leading the program. Interestingly, one experimental study found that while white women are often penalized for having dominant leadership styles, Asian American women are not (Tinkler, Zhao, Li, & Ridgeway, 2019). The authors argue that it may simply be because people do not remember the details of Asian women's actual behavior due to their intersectional invisibility, whereas they are more likely to scrutinize white women's behavior (Tinkler et al., 2019). I remember one judgment error that I made early in my program director role. In the heat of the moment when dealing with an urgent matter, I inadvertently ignored the proper procedures and made a request to senior administration on behalf of the program. Later, I learned that the head of another unit, a white man, who went along with my idea and made a similar demand for his unit, got into trouble with senior administration, even though I was the one who initiated the behavior. I also noticed that people would often tell me that I am polite, nice, and nonconfrontational, even after they witnessed me being assertive. It seems those nonstereotypical behaviors do not register in peoples' minds.

With my visibility as program director, I am often invited to participate in events, give talks, or join committees under the umbrella of equity, diversity, and inclusion. Soon after I took my current position, I was invited to join university-wide committees one after another. I was flattered by these invitations initially, and at the same time, puzzled by them. I did not know how I was selected from everyone in the community. After attending the first meetings, I quickly gathered that I was probably invited to join the committees because of aspect(s) of identity that I bring to the table. I appreciated these committees recognizing the importance of being more inclusive and having voices from diverse groups. However, I felt out of place attending the meetings because I was invited as a representative of one (or two, or three) underrepresented groups, and there were few (if any) people like me at the table. Tokenism that faculties of color experience has been documented both in Canada and the USA (Henry & Tator, 2012; Settles, Buchanan, & Dotson, 2019). Ahmed (2012) writes, "People of color are welcomed on condition they return that hospitality by integrating into a common organizational culture, or by 'being' diverse, and allowing in situations to celebrate their diversity" (p. 43). Minority faculties' passion to help and support their own and other communities align conveniently with this institutional agenda. Faculty women of color are "extreme tokens" (Turner et al., 2011, p. 207) who are "overburdened by service demands" (Hirshfield &

Joseph, 2012, p. 220). As a nontenured faculty with enormous administrative responsibilities, I had to learn to say no to these invitations, no matter how much I cared about the causes.

I Am Here!

Asian Americans and Asian Canadians (including East Asian, South Asian, and Southeast Asian) made up of 7% and 14% of the total USA and Canadian populations, respectively, according to the most recent census data (Statistics Canada, 2017). Despite high educational achievement as a group, Asians in North America are often seen as great workers, but not leaders (Kawahara et al., 2013; Sanchez-Hucles & Davis, 2010; Sy, Tram-Quon, & Leung, 2017). The majority of university senior administrators in the USA, except chief diversity officers, are white. Asian Americans hold between 1% and 3% of senior administration positions (depending on the job), following Blacks (5–13%) and Hispanics (2–6%) (Nixon, 2017). Comparing women and men, Asian American women are perceived less fit for leadership than Asian American men (Tinkler et al., 2019). Contrary to the myth of the model minority, it is clear that Asians contend with "bamboo ceiling" (Hyun, 2012). There are a number of common Asian values, beliefs, and practices that are in direct conflict with the values, beliefs, and practices that are perceived important for leadership in North America (Kawahara et al., 2013; Sanchez-Hucles & Davis, 2010; Sy et al., 2017). My culture taught me not to stand out, not to take up space, and to prioritize others' needs over my own. Typical of Asians, I was also taught that there is no need to ask for a raise and promotion because the boss will recognize good work and give us what we deserve (Kawahara et al., 2013; Sanchez-Hucles & Davis, 2010; Sy et al., 2017); of course we never know when we will be recognized or if we actually will be recognized. Having lived in North America for nearly 30 years, I have learned that I have to find a way to take up space when the opportunities are presented, without losing myself and my culture. As a queer woman of color with some power, it is my responsibility to take up space and sit at the table so that more of us will be at the table and change the statistics. I must continue to try to break the bamboo ceiling.

My leadership style is similar to my therapy model that is based on the Japanese understanding of self, called "jibun." In Japanese culture, self is one's share of the whole, and individuals in any relationship are sharing physical and emotional space (Taniguchi, 2005). I believe one of my roles as a therapist is to open up space for my clients so that they can have as much space as they need in the relationship with me. Similarly, one of the major roles in leadership positions is to create space for others, especially those who are on the margins, so they can have their share or "jibun." The simplest and hardest way for me to do that is to "show up" because I know that people with multiple-marginalized identities can create space with their presence (Nixon, 2017), and I feel a responsibility to do that. The isolation that women faculty of color experience is well documented (Nixon, 2017; Sanchez-Hucles &

Davis, 2010; Turner et al., 2011). Imagine arriving at an event or meeting alone, finding nobody who looks like you, and feeling totally out of place. Showing up is a simple act but can be very difficult. Now, imagine you are a person of color or a queer person who finds me smiling at you at an event. One of the advantages of belonging to several underrepresented groups is that by being present, I can potentially create exponentially more space than people with single marginalities. This act of showing up is a first-order change that may or may not elicit change in the system. When the system is rigid, opening up space for some means yielding space for others. This often triggers resentment for those who have to give up some of their space. Space remains a manifestation of patriarchy, white supremacy, homophobia, transphobia, ableism, xenophobia, etc. My responsibility as a leader, therefore, is to respectfully demand that the system expand and grow so that individuals from underrepresented groups will not only show up, but also stay in the space.

I can think of moments when I attempted to create space for others using my power. The examples are focused on Indigenous communities because decolonization in Canada is currently centered around Indigenous and non-Indigenous relations. Upon my arrival to the program, I noticed that the curriculum did not include any Indigenous-focused courses, and there were no Indigenous instructors or supervisors. In fact, all instructors and supervisors were white. I realized that it was going to take some time to develop relationships with Indigenous people and/or communities, recruit instructors/supervisors, and develop an Indigenous-focused MFT course. While I worked on building relationships, as program director, I asked all existing course instructors to include Indigenous content in their courses as a first step.

There was an opportunity to facilitate a panel discussion on Indigenous perspectives at an event. I consulted with some Indigenous students in the program, and we organized a panel discussion, where those students shared their experiences of going through colonial MFT education and training. Students told me they were unhappy with a major change the event organizers suggested to the title, and I supported them in resisting. It was isomorphic that a group of settlers tried to tell Indigenous students what title they should use to describe their own experiences. I also told the student panelists that they did not have to conduct the conversation in a colonial way if they did not want to, which was my attempt to open up space for them. During another event after one of the keynote addresses, I noticed one white person from the audience was talking to the Indigenous keynote speaker for a long time. It was clear to me that the person had no awareness of the amount of space that they were taking at an event that the Indigenous speaker created mostly for people in their community. I then noticed that a student of color was standing in line patiently waiting for her turn. Using my power, I decided to politely interrupt the monologue and made the attendee aware of the others' existence in the space.

These are things I may not have been able to do if I was not a program director. They are small examples of the way I was able to use my power and create space for others who are also marginalized. Ever since I began working as MFT program director in my current university, three white women, including one queer woman, took me under their wing. They were all powerful women with senior administrative positions. Women faculty of color in leadership do not normally have access to informal networks or the old boys' club, in which insiders receive information and support to help them navigate the system (Sanchez-Hucles & Davis, 2010). Even as a regular faculty member, it was clear that I did not have access to this type of network. As a queer immigrant Asian woman who is in a leadership position, having these three women's mentorship has been crucial in navigating the unfamiliar system. They have all stood up for me when needed. They certainly created space for me.

Having lived in Canada and USA, I think that the countries are more different than Americans want to believe, and more similar than Canadians want to believe. In Canada, there is an umbrella federal law to prohibit discrimination based on "race, national or ethnic origin, color, religion, age, sex, sexual orientation, gender identity or expression, marital status, family status, genetic characteristics, disability and conviction for an offence for which a pardon has been granted or in respect of which a record suspension has been ordered" (Canadian Human Rights Act, R.S.C., 1985, c. H-6). In spite of this law, discriminations and violence against these groups and individuals exist in Canada too. Systemic and institutional inequalities are prominent, and certain groups of people benefit from them while others are disadvantaged. Boyko (1998) argues that Canada has climbed up all rungs of the "racist ladder" from stereotypes to genocide (p. 11). Having this law in place, however, makes me feel empowered and less frightened when I decide to challenge systems for manifesting identity-based discrimination, because the law says it is wrong, period.

In this chapter, I discussed the dimensions of race and gender more than sexual orientation. Because my queerness is invisible, it is difficult to identify its unique impact on my professional relationships. It is important that I am "out" as program director because my queerness opens up space for those who identify as queer, two two spirit, or LGBT. Research suggests that queers who are able to integrate their sexuality with their professional identity perceive their work environment more positively and engage in relational leadership styles (Henderson, Simon, & Henicheck, 2018). There are several themes related to sexual orientation that go beyond this chapter. Whether or not my queerness helps or hinders my position as program director is unknown. In reflecting on this chapter, I wonder if my queerness helps me escape some Asian women stereotypes (passivity, obedience, and eroticization) that are not considered suitable for leadership. Exploration of queer-focused themes would be a fruitful future endeavor.

My experience of being an MFT program director is unique to me but may be familiar to some others. I certainly hope that sharing my experience opens up some space for readers. I am always in awe when I reflect on my life's journey. Look at me! A Japanese girl who was told by her father that she did not have to go to university because she is a girl is now a program director at a Canadian university and living my father's dream of making a name and doing business globally. Confusion Corner still confuses and frightens me at times, but I know I can always ask my mentors to help me navigate. I am going to continue taking up space as often as I can, respectfully demanding that systems expand and grow, and opening space for others who, like me, are underrepresented in academia.

Acknowledgment This chapter would not have existed without my partner, Jane, who lives for conversations about white supremacy, patriarchy, misogyny, hegemony, colonialism, nationalism, and/or neoliberalism, who encourages me to take up space while respecting my values of silence and humility, and understands my fear of standing out.

References

Ahmed, S. (2012). *On being included: Racism and diversity in institutional life*. Durham, NC: Duke University Press.

Ayman, R., & Korabik, K. (2010). Leadership: Why gender and culture matter. *American Psychologist, 65*(3), 157–170. https://doi.org/10.1037/a0018806.

Bertalanffy, L. (1969). *General system theory: Foundations, development, applications*. New York, NY: George Braziller.

Bishop, A. (2015). *Becoming an ally: Breaking the cycle of oppression in people* (3rd ed.). Black Point, NS: Fernwood Publishing.

Boyko, J. (1998). *Last steps to freedom: The evolution of Canadian racism*. Winnipeg, MB: J. Gordon Shillingford Pub.

Canadian Human Rights Act, R.S.C. (1985). c. H-6, s. 3 1996, c. 14, s. 2 2012, c. 1, s. 138(E) 2017, c. 3, ss. 10, 11, c. 13, s. 2. Retrieved from the Justice Laws website: https://laws-lois.justice.gc.ca/eng/acts/h-6/index.html.

Crenshaw, K. (1989). Demarginalizing the intersection of race and sex: A Black feminist critique of antidiscrimination doctrine, feminist theory and antiracist politics. *University of Chicago Legal Forum, 1989*. Retrieved from https://chicagounbound.uchicago.edu/uclf/vol1989/iss1/8.

D'Arrigo-Patrick, J., Hoff, C., Knudson-Martin, C., & Tuttle, A. (2017). Navigating critical theory and postmodernism: Social justice and therapist power in family therapy. *Family Process, 56*(3), 574–588. https://doi.org/10.1111/famp.12236.

Eng, D. L., Halberstam, J., & Muñoz, J. E. (2005). Introduction. *Social Text, 23*(3–4 (84–85)), 1–17. https://doi.org/10.1215/01642472-23-3-4_84-85-1.

Hashimoto, G. E. (2012). --Nisei--Sansei--Yonsei--: Intergenerational communication of the Internment and the lived experience of twelve Japanese Canadians born after the Internment. Master's thesis, University of Manitoba, Manitoba, Canada. Retrieved from https://primo-pmtna01.hosted.exlibrisgroup.com/permalink/f/1q3bkt5/UMB_ALMA21546439470001651.

Henderson, M. M., Simon, K. A., & Henicheck, J. (2018). The relationship between sexuality–professional identity integration and leadership in the workplace. *Psychology of Sexual Orientation and Gender Diversity, 5*(3), 338–351. https://doi.org/10.1037/sgd0000277.

Henry, F., & Tator, C. (2012). Interviews with racialized faculty members in Canadian universities. *Canadian Ethnic Studies, 44*(2), 75–99. https://doi.org/10.1353/ces.2012.0003.

Hirshfield, L. E., & Joseph, T. D. (2012). 'We need a woman, we need a black woman': Gender, race, and identity taxation in the academy. *Gender & Education, 24*(2), 213–227. https://doi.org/10.1080/09540253.2011.606208.

Hyun, J. (2012). Leadership principles for capitalizing on culturally diverse teams: The bamboo ceiling revisited. *Leader to Leader, 2012*(64), 14–19. https://doi.org/10.1002/ltl.20017.

Kawahara, D. M., Pal, M. S., & Chin, J. L. (2013). The leadership experiences of Asian Americans. *Asian American Journal of Psychology, 4*(4), 240–248. https://doi.org/10.1037/a0035196.

Moody, J. (2011). *Faculty diversity: Removing the barriers*. New York, NY: Routledge.

Nagata, D. K., Kim, J. H. J., & Nguyen, T. U. (2015). Processing cultural trauma: Intergenerational effects of the Japanese American incarceration. *Journal of Social Issues, 71*(2), 356–370. https://doi.org/10.1111/josi.12115.

Nixon, M. L. (2017). Experiences of women of color university chief diversity officers. *Journal of Diversity in Higher Education, 10*(4), 301–317. https://doi.org/10.1037/dhe0000043.

Purdie-Vaughns, V., & Eibach, R. P. (2008). Intersectional invisibility: The distinctive advantages and disadvantages of multiple subordinate-group identities. *Sex Roles, 59*(5), 377–391. https://doi.org/10.1007/s11199-008-9424-4.

Sanchez-Hucles, J. V., & Davis, D. D. (2010). Women and women of color in leadership: Complexity, identity, and intersectionality. *American Psychologist, 65*(3), 171–181. https://doi.org/10.1037/a0017459.

Settles, I. H., Buchanan, N. T., & Dotson, K. (2019). Scrutinized but not recognized: (In)visibility and hypervisibility experiences of faculty of color. *Journal of Vocational Behavior, 113*, 62–74. https://doi.org/10.1016/j.jvb.2018.06.003.

Statistics Canada. (2017). Census Profile, 2016 Census. [Catalogue no. 98-316-X2016001]. Retrieved from Statistics Canada website: https://www12.statcan.gc.ca/census-recensement/2016/dp-pd/prof/index.cfm?Lang=E.

Sy, T., Tram-Quon, S., & Leung, A. (2017). Developing minority leaders: Key success factors of Asian Americans. *Asian American Journal of Psychology, 8*(2), 142–155. https://doi.org/10.1037/aap0000075.

Taniguchi, N. (2005). From polarization to pluralization: The Japanese sense of self and Bowen theory. In M. Rastogi & E. Wieling (Eds.), *Voices of color: First-person accounts of ethnic minority therapists* (pp. 265–276). Thousand Oaks, CA: Sage Publications. https://doi.org/10.4135/9781452231662.n15.

Tinkler, J., Zhao, J., Li, Y., & Ridgeway, C. L. (2019). Honorary whites? Asian American women and the dominance penalty. *Socius: Sociological Research for a Dynamic World, 5*, 1–13. https://doi.org/10.1177/2378023119836000.

Turner, C. S. V., González, J. C., & Wong (Lau), K. (2011). Faculty women of color: The critical nexus of race and gender. *Journal of Diversity in Higher Education, 4*(4), 199–211. https://doi.org/10.1037/a0024630.

Wieling, E., Negretti, M. A., Stokes, S., Kimball, T., Christensen, F. B., & Bryan, L. (2001). Postmodernism in marriage and family therapy training: Doctoral students' understanding and experiences. *Journal of Marital and Family Therapy, 27*(4), 527–533. https://doi.org/10.1111/j.1752-0606.2001.tb00345.x.

Chapter 5
"*Sí, Se Puede Educar*": Impacts on the Classroom Environment from the Perspective of a US-Born, Latino Male, Religious Minority Faculty

Sergio B. Pereyra

The Spanish phrase "*Sí, se puede*" was coined by Latina/o activists Dolores Huerta and Cesar Chavez. When translated in the correct context, it means "Yes, it can be done." This inspiring motto helped unite Latino/a migrant farm workers in California's Central Valley and Arizona in the fight against exploitation, unfair wages and horrendous work conditions. This phrase has not only been adopted by other civil and labor rights Latino groups around the country, but it has also been transformed to create new meaning for the children of those migrant farm workers who are searching for a better education, many of whom have made their way into my classroom. The Spanish word "*educar*" means "to teach" or "to educate," but its scope is more social than academic. The Latino cultural value of "*educación*" or "*ser bien educado*" (depicted in the literature as "*ser buen educado*," but corrected grammatically in Spanish here) connotes being well-mannered, respectful and having high morals (Turcios-Cotto & Milan, 2013). From my lens as an educator, the combination of these two terms signifies an empowering responsibility to not only teach aspiring Marriage and Family Therapy (MFT) clinical skills, but also to encourage the underrepresented, to educate students about social justice issues and to help students learn how to respect and even positively esteem those who are different from them.

This chapter is about my experiences as a tenure-track faculty at Fresno State University. I will describe the social location of my macrosystem and ecosystems (department and classroom) while taking into account a Latina/o critical race theory perspective (Irizarry, 2012) and will then describe the changes I have experienced with my development over time as a Fresno State faculty. In addition, I will discuss the social interactions in my social location and describe how I use my power to

S. B. Pereyra (✉)
Marriage and Family Therapy Program, Fresno State University, Fresno, CA, USA
e-mail: spereyra@csufresno.edu; spereyra@mail.fresnostate.edu

© Springer Nature Switzerland AG 2021   43
K. M.-T. Quek, A. L. Hsieh (eds.), *Intersectionality in Family Therapy Leadership*, AFTA SpringerBriefs in Family Therapy,
https://doi.org/10.1007/978-3-030-67977-4_5

influence my students. Lastly, I will share what I feel needs to change in the education system in order to account for my cultural-social location.

While this chapter focuses on issues and experiences from a Latino perspective, it should be noted that the choice in the term "Latino/a" is used very deliberately. The term "Latinx" has grown and gained lots of popularity in different fields in the social sciences and education; while I empathize with the "Latinx" movement to challenge the male dominance of the Latino culture and to be more inclusive of LGBTQ individuals (deOnís, 2017), the "Latinx" term does not represent my personal experience as a Latino male with stronger ties to my Mexican and Argentine heritage. To me, the term "Latinx" is an anglicization of my beautiful, native Spanish language and represents another form of colonization in the linguistic sense. In my experience, the term "Latinx" is completely incomprehensible to most Latino/as outside the USA, and I would prefer to give preference to the more marginalized Latino immigrant group than to the more privileged US-born Latinos who insist on the Americanized term. I have no problem using the term with those "Latinx" individuals who choose it for themselves but would also like the same consideration and choice and would not like to be lumped into that label.

Eco-developmental Theoretical Framework

Eco-Developmental theory—an integration of Bronfenbrenner's ecological systems theory (1979) and classical developmental theory (e.g., Braveman & Barclay, 2009)—has been useful in describing experiences of Latinos in the USA, in previous literature (Prado et al., 2010). Consequently, Latino/a experiences are influenced by the interacting elements of the individual's ecosystem, development over time and social interactions (Prado & Pantin, 2011). The two main ecosystems relevant to my experience with regard to my social location are the microsystem, depicting the influences of my family, church community and school, and the macrosystem, which comprises my cultural experience and the sociopolitical climate of the USA. Changes in my cultural and professional development over time will be presented, and the social interactions that have most shaped my social location in my role as an educator at Fresno State University is discussed.

Identity as a US-Born Religious Minority and Latino Male

Even though I was born in the USA, I identify as a Mexican Argentine and not as an American. My father is from Argentina and my mother is from Mexico. While the Spanish language was my first language, it quickly became dominated by the English language due to microsystemic influences (e.g., school, friends, television, etc.) in my early childhood. I was born in Provo, Utah, but I was raised in Houston, Texas, which I still consider my home and where I come from. Like so many other

Mexican Americans, I too felt that I was not Mexican enough to be accepted by the Latinos in my community, and simultaneously, I felt rejected by those who challenged my "Americanness" based on the color of my skin and Latino features. But most of the ethnic discrimination I have personally experienced has been at the hands of police officers. While it is beyond the scope of this chapter to recount the many negative experiences I have had as a male of color with police officers, it is sufficient to say that I am still extremely triggered and have real visceral reactions when I see police officers, especially with their flashing lights.

The importance of spirituality is a very commonly held cultural value among many Latinos (Falicov, 1998); my family was no different in that regard. However, my family veered from the stereotypical Catholic background that so many other Latinos cling to. I am a member of the Church of Jesus Christ of Latter-day Saints. People might be more aware of the nickname given to us by others—"Mormons"— but it should be noted that we are not the "Mormon Church"; that church does not exist. Growing up in the South, I remember feeling like I had to defend my faith against many who believed that we were a cult or a sect and not even really Christian. I guess this is part of the reason Russell M. Nelson, president of the Church of Jesus Christ of Latter-day Saints, publicly made an announcement reaffirming the actual name of our church and asking members and nonmembers alike to refrain from referring to us as "Mormons" (Weaver, 2018). The Church of Jesus Christ (acceptable abbreviation; Weaver, 2018) has also received a lot of criticism from people who say that it is a US- (and particularly White-) dominated religion. However, people might not realize that since the year 2000, there are now more members of the Church of Jesus Christ of Latter-day Saints outside than inside the USA, and that Spanish, not English, is the most widely spoken language in the Church today (Todd, 2000). Much of my "*educación*" (Turcios-Cotto & Milan, 2013) comes from this religious perspective.

Scholars have historically tried to understand Latino culture and parse out gender roles according to their own perceptions; within those perceptions, Latino males have been labeled with the term "machismo" (Ingoldsby, 2006; Moreno, 2007). Aggression, excessive drinking (alcohol), violence, hypersexuality and promiscuity have been prominent embodiments of this term throughout the literature (Ingoldsby, 2006; Moreno, 2007). For example, Ingoldsby (2006) stated, "… the preferred goal is the conquest of many women. To take advantage of a young woman sexually is cause for pride and prestige, not blame, and some men will commit adultery just to prove to themselves that they can do it. Excepting the wife and a mistress, long term affectionate relationships should not exist. Sexual conquests are to satisfy male vanity. Indeed, one's potency must be known by others, which leads to bragging and storytelling. A married man should have a mistress in addition to casual encounters. His relationship with his wife is that of an aloof lord-protector" (p. 282).

These degrading and destructive narratives are extremely offensive to me. Unfortunately, the Latina female gender role is not much more favorably described in the literature; Latina women are often characterized as being weak, submissive, subservient and self-sacrificing through the term "marianismo" (Ingoldsby, 2006; Moreno, 2007). But if this is the rhetoric that service providers and educators are ascribing to, then it would make perfect sense why Latinos are underserved and even discriminated against by those service providers and educators (e.g., Irizarry, 2012). I feel like I have spent a great deal of time fighting against negative perceptions and stereotypes of Latinos, and Latino men in particular, all my life. As a licensed clinician and an educator in a MFT training program, I have strived to challenge those assumptions and pretenses and replace them with ones that are more conducive to serving Latinos (Falicov, 2010).

The Ecosystem of My Current Social Location

After completing my doctoral degree from Brigham Young University (BYU), I accepted a tenure-track position as an assistant professor at California State University, Fresno (more commonly known as Fresno State University or FSU). Fresno, California, is a diverse city with a high concentration of Latino/a migrant farm workers, many of whom are undocumented. My career at Fresno State started around the same time that Donald Trump was running for president of the USA. I remember seeing his anti-immigrant and anti-Latino propaganda and thought in my mind that no reasonable US citizen would really vote for him. I was dumbfounded and shocked when he actually won the election. In that moment, the US flag morphed from a symbol of freedom into a symbol of oppression and intolerance to me. I started my faculty position in this tense and adversarial macrosystem at Fresno State University. From an eco-developmental perspective (Prado et al., 2010), I was expecting that the shift in my microsystem—that is, coming from a more homogenous environment in Utah, where I completed my graduate work, to Fresno, California, where more people looked and spoke like me (Latino/as)—would be an "easier" shift, but it was not. The "*Sí, se puede*" motto was put to test.

When Trump became president, there was a drastic decline in the number of Latino clients seeking treatment at our very own Fresno family counseling center, which is where our graduate students receive their practicum hours. I remember many Fresno State students crying and worrying, fearing the disruption of their families and the deportation of their parents. But I also remember, insensitive White students in Make America Great Again (MAGA) attire harassing, taunting and belittling other Latino students. On one occasion, Fresno State held a celebration to honor the statewide holiday Cesar Chavez Day, which is observed in memory of the Central Valley native Latino who cocreated the "*Sí, se puede*" motto. This celebration was disrupted by Trump-supporting Fresno State students who rudely interjected and protested, expressing anti-Latino and anti-immigrant sentiments during the celebration. It caused enough of a scene to prompt the president of Fresno State University to make a public statement affirming freedom of speech, while also condemning this lack of "*educación*" (Turcios-Cotto & Milan, 2013) and reiterating a campus culture of inclusion. While I was used to the microaggressions and subtle oppression of Latino students in educational microsystems (Irizarry, 2012; Turcios-Cotto & Milan, 2013), I had to learn how to respond to more blatant forms of oppression against Latinos under the magnifying glass of other young Latino students looking to me for guidance due to the polarized macrosystem. I was put in a unique position of power as a Latino educator with the highest level of education in a predominately Latino campus community.

In the ecosystem of my classroom, I am very aware of my power and privilege not only as the instructor, but also as a US-born cisgender male. Similar to critical race theory (Bell, 1980), Latina/o critical race theory (LatCrit) analyzes phenomena in terms of race, while including intersections of other factors, such as gender, ethnicity, immigration status, religion, language, etc., which more adequately represent the experience of Latinos in the USA (Irizarry, 2012). In a sense, LatCrit "challenges the Black/White binary that often limits considerations of race and racism to two groups, thereby creating discursive space for Latinos/as who can be of any race and individuals who may be multiracial" (Irizarry, 2012, p. 293).

From a LatCrit perspective, I can think of two specific ways that my presence as a person in power can alter the classroom environment. First, as one who has known discrimination through more than one aspect (ethnicity, religion, etc.), I am more open to the unique oppressive experiences of others that might go beyond race. I am willing to validate those oppressive experiences and teach students to validate those kinds of experiences for their clients. Second, as one who has had issues with authority, I am open to feedback as the authority figure in the classroom and encourage students to challenge authority when they feel they are wronged.

My Development Over Time in My Social Location

My upbringing and personal experiences of oppression would come to impact my response to my ecosystem, but my development as a professional educator also underwent great change, especially in terms of power. Though a brand-new faculty to Fresno State, I was used to the academic rigor of a research university because of my experiences at BYU, and I was quickly branded by my students as the "hard professor." After much reflection and some great mentoring from senior Fresno State faculty, I changed my approach and "eased up" on some of my expectations for my students, and I started getting a better feel for the Fresno State student ecosystem and macrosystem.

I experienced another developmental change in regards to the faculty ecosystem. Like other new faculty experiences, my first year was marked by much stress, confusion and powerlessness (Austin, 2003), especially related to our governing accreditation and enmeshed department. I was coming from a COAMFTE- (MFT-specific) accredited institution into a CACREP- (LPC-specific) accredited institution. Even though the California professional licensure uses the language "Licensed Marriage and Family Therapist" (LMFT), I had to get used to using the CACREP language of "counselor"; our program is called "Marriage, Family, and Child Counseling" (MFCC). It didn't (and still does not) make sense to me why our program is CACREP-accredited and not COAMFTE-accredited. When I raised that particular question, I received no real explanation and was even met with hostility. Our department comprises a school counseling (K-12) program, student affairs and college counseling (SACC) program, rehabilitation counseling program and our MFCC program. Most of the "core" courses are offered to students from all four programs, which lead to some confusion among the students regarding scope of competence and scope of practice. But even with this intermingling, I remember a faculty from another department explicitly saying that our MFCC program and their program are inherently at a turf war, which added to the stressful departmental microsystem.

After 4 years, I have now come to terms with the CACREP accreditation and have learned to better navigate the other struggles mentioned by taking advantage of good mentoring and faculty peer-support systems like other faculty of color (Cole, McGowan, & Zerquera, 2017), even though I have not felt a change in my power-lessness as a junior faculty, especially regarding our department policy and procedures.

The last change I have experienced based on my social location has been the most rewarding to me. Growing up as a Christian, I cannot deny the homophobia I was taught and was socialized to internalize. I particularly remembered feeling scared that one of my gay clients would become attracted to me and would try to change the therapeutic relationship into a sexual one. After much education, strug-gle and maturity, I can now happily say that I have changed my homophobic ways and now consider myself an LGBTQ ally. Ironically, I have now become a lot more leery of having people learn that I am a member of the Church of Jesus Christ, espe-cially in California, where LGBTQ issues are always at the forefront of cultural sensitivity. But after feeling more comfortable with my multicultural class, I decided to come out to them as a "Mormon." Students have shared their difficulty in under-standing how I can be such an advocate for LGBTQ issues in one-class session, and then in another confess that I am a member of a very conservative church, although I would not consider myself to be a "conservative" or "liberal" (none of these fit with my experience).

While it is true that my religion teaches that acting out homosexually is a sin (but not identifying as someone with same-gender attraction), it also teaches us that we all sin, God is the only one that has a right to judge us for any sins, and to love one another (Matthew 22:39, New Testament; 3 Nephi 12:43–44, Book of Mormon; Doctrine & Covenants 59:6). I tell my confused students that I love my LGBTQ "neighbors" just as much as myself and empathize with their pain, and that I do not need to concern myself with their sexual identity or orientation, unless they need me as an advocate. This gives religious students hope and encouragement and inspires the "*Sí, se puede*" attitude in other meaningful ways in a safe classroom ecosystem. I completely understand that many LGBTQ individuals have most likely experi-enced dreadful oppression from members of my church. I don't feel bad when they might not readily trust me after learning that I graduated from BYU (a private church-educational institution), but I am happy when they do give me a chance to show them a different experience as a member of the Church of Jesus Christ of Latter-day Saints.

Social Interactions in My Social Location

From an eco-developmental perspective, social interactions become a prominent feature in the meaning-making of experiences for Latinos (Prado et al., 2010). This is also in line with macrosystemic influences of "personalismo," which is a Latino cultural value highlighting the importance that Latinos place on interpersonal inter-action, warmth and trust (Falicov, 1998; Leidy, Guerra, & Toro, 2010). My relation-ship with my students is very important to me; I make it a point to learn and remember each student's name and to give them positive encouragement when par-ticipating in class, especially those from marginalized groups. My own cultural background influences this interaction as well. As a Mexican Argentine who is proud of his cultural heritage, I encourage other minorities to be proud of the diver-sity they bring into the classroom. I encourage a *"Sí, se puede"* attitude of learning in the classroom and look for ways to not only teach the secular material needed as an MFT, but also the *"educación"* (Turcios-Cotto & Milan, 2013) that extends beyond the classroom, mostly by my own example.

In terms of how students might respond to me based on my social identities, I can think of two different experiences. As a "Hispanic-serving institution," we are for-tunate to have a very high number of Latino students in our programs. In this aspect, my experience in my social interactions with students has been quite positive, as other Latino students have expressed the way they look up to me as a role model. This is most likely amplified, given the many disparities Latinos face in education, such as high dropout rates, low representation in higher education and lower aca-demic performance (Hill & Torres, 2010). I use my power to encourage my Latino students to openly challenge these disparities and to challenge the power structures of higher education that discourage bilingualism, that are insensitive to undocu-mented immigrants and their personal situations and that fail to provide adequate resources for Latino parents who do not speak English. In addition, I encourage students to challenge the pernicious presidential propaganda so widely promoted in our sociopolitical macrosystem.

I also try to use my position of power to open up space for my more privileged students to engage in difficult conversations, to reflect on their own privilege and to challenge the "meritocracy" narrative most of them have been led to believe (Tatum, 2003). This is particularly relevant in the multicultural counseling course I teach. In my social interactions with them, I try to lead by example in describing all of the "unmerited" benefits I receive just by being a US-born heterosexual cisgender male. But many of my more privileged students seem to struggle most when we go over nationalism, which is such an under-addressed topic in MFT programs even in mul-ticultural education (Platt & Laszloffy, 2013). I also think that the current macrosys-tem of my social location makes it easier to confuse patriotism with nationalism. Patriotism is a devotion of country and a desire for the country to be the best it can be, while nationalism is the belief that ones' own country is superior to all others and that its interests are far more important than those of any other country (Primoratz, 2009). As Platt and Laszloffy (2013) so eloquently state, "Just as with the other 'isms' (i.e., racism, sexism, ableism, lookism), nationalism lends itself to patterns of domination and polarization and therefore, like the other 'isms' it is important to recognize and confront manifestations of nationalism" (p. 443). This is slightly different from ethnocentrism, which is more of a belief that your ethnicity (not necessarily country) is better than everyone else's. Some of my students struggle with the cognitive dissonance of believing that this is the greatest country in the world but also witnessing how this government put undocumented Latino immigrant children in cages after running out of room in detention facilities.

The last social interaction that has impacted my current social location circles back to my experiences with other faculty. As mentioned previously, much of what is presumed about Latino "maleness" comes from literature that depicts us as domineering, hypersexual and overpowering (Ingoldsby, 2006). I have tried to show others a different picture. While I feel I have been more successful among my students, I have had less luck among some of my colleagues. One of our responsibilities as a tenure-track faculty is to provide peer evaluations for adjunct faculty. During an evaluation with one particular adjunct (whose identifiers will be omitted for confidentiality), I tried to be as honest and unbiased as possible and frankly felt that her lesson was unacceptable. During my write-up, I not only included very specific feedback on the things I felt were lacking and how she could improve them, but I also shared a few pieces of encouragement and things that she did well. However, during the social interaction of the debriefing, she responded with a lot of reactivity, hostility and sexism. In her official written response, she continued confirming the negative "male" Latino narrative by stating that I was "chauvinistic, domineering and arrogant." I could understand her disappointment and frustration for receiving her first negative evaluation, but I was trying to be honest and professional, and I think that her additive "machista" comments were unnecessary.

Changes to Account for My Cultural-Social Location

In closing, I feel that there is a lot that needs to change in the education system in order to account for my cultural-social location, but I will only share one idea. From a LatCrit perspective (Irizarry, 2012), educators and administrators need to be sensitive not only to how power differentials are manifested through race, but also through other nuanced cultural factors, such as immigration status, ethnicity and so forth. In order to account for my cultural-social location, challenges need to be made to the concept of "cultural competence." It is "a myth that is typically American and located in the metaphor of American 'know-how.' It is consistent with the belief that knowledge brings control and effectiveness, and that this is an ideal to be achieved above all else. I question the notion that one could become 'competent' at the culture of another" (Dean, 2001, p. 624). I echo that sentiment and would add that when students feel that they "learn enough" (definition of competence) about a culture, they tend to prescribe more, overgeneralize, label, stereotype and run the risk of misunderstanding—or worse, invalidating—another's cultural experience. I endorse taking an "informed not-knowing stance," which means that one still strives to educate themselves about other cultures and remains continually open to new knowledge, especially when received directly from their own clients about their own culture (Dean, 2001). *"Sí, se puede"* (we can) make changes when we have the heart and willingness to do so.

Acknowledgments First and foremost, I would like to thank my loving Father in heaven and my Savior, Lord and Redeemer, Jesus Christ. I would also like to acknowledge the love of my life, my wife, Raquel, without whose support none of this would be possible. Next, I would like to mention my pride and joy, my sons, Sinaí and Alema, and *"mi corazón,"* my daughter, Adaia. I also want to thank my parents and my siblings who have contributed most to my growth and development. Additionally, I would like to thank my master's program mentor, Dr. Jonathan Sandberg, and my doctoral program mentor, Dr. Roy Bean. Lastly, I would like to thank my work companion, peer and friend, Dr. Jeff Crane, and my Fresno State University mentor, Dr. Kyle Weir, for his great support and mentorship.

References

Austin, A. E. (2003). Creating a bridge to the future: Preparing new faculty to face changing expectations in a shifting context. *The Review of Higher Education, 26*(2), 119–144.

Bell, D. (1980). *Race, racism and American law*. Boston, MA: Little, Brown.

Braveman, P., & Barclay, C. (2009). Health disparities beginning in childhood: A life-course perspective. *Pediatrics, 124*, 163–175.

Bronfenbrenner, U. (1979). Contexts of child rearing: Problems and prospects. *American Psychologist, 34*, 844–850.

Cole, E. R., McGowan, B. L., & Zerquera, D. D. (2017). First-year faculty of color: Narratives about entering the academy. *Equity & Excellence in Education, 50*(1), 1–12.

Dean, R. G. (2001). The myth of cross-cultural competence. *Families in Society, 82*(6), 623–630.

deOnís. (2017). What's in an "x"? An exchange about the politics of "Latinx". *Chiricú Journal, 1*(32), 78–91.

Falicov, C. J. (1998). *Latino families in therapy: A guide to multicultural practice*. New York, NY: Guilford.

Falicov, C. J. (2010). Changing constructions of machismo for Latino men in therapy: The devil never sleeps. *Family Process, 49*, 309–329.

Hill, N. E., & Torres, K. (2010). Negotiating the American Dream: The paradox of aspirations and achievement among Latino students and engagement between their families and schools. *Journal of Social Issues, 66*(1), 95–112.

Ingoldsby, B. (2006). Families in Latin America. In B. B. Ingoldsby & S. D. Smith (Eds.), *Families in global and multicultural perspective* (pp. 274–290). Thousand Oaks, CA: Sage Publications.

Irizarry, J. G. (2012). Los caminos: Latino/a youth forging pathways in pursuit of higher education. *Journal of Hispanic Higher Education, 11*(3), 291–309.

Leidy, M., Guerra, N., & Toro, R. (2010). A review of family-based programs to prevent youth violence among Latinos. *Hispanic Journal of Behavioral Sciences, 32*(1), 5–36.

Moreno, C. L. (2007). The relationship between culture, gender, structural factors, abuse, trauma, and HIV/AIDS for Latinas. *Qualitative Health Research, 17*(3), 340–352.

Platt, J. J., & Laszloffy, T. A. (2013). Critical patriortism: Incorporating nationality into MFT education and training. *Journal of Marital and Family Therapy, 39*(4), 441–456.

Prado, G., Huang, S., Maldonado-Molina, M., Bandiera, F., Schwartz, S. J., de la Vega, P., et al. (2010). An empirical test of eco-developmental theory in predicting HIV risk behaviors among Hispanic youth. *Health Education & Behavior, 37*(1), 97–114.

Prado, G., & Pantin, H. (2011). Reducing substance use and HIV health disparities among Hispanic youth in the USA: The Familias Unidas program of research. *Psychosocial Intervention, 20*(1), 63–73.

Primoratz, I. (2009). Patriotism. In E. N. Zalta (Ed.), *The Stanford encyclopedia of philosophy.* Retrieved from http://plato.stanford.edu/archives/sum2009/entries/patriotism/

Tatum, B. D. (2003). *"Why are all the Black kids sitting together in the cafeteria?": And other conversations about race.* New York, NY: Basic Books.

Todd, J. M. (2000). *Historic Milestone Achieved: More Non-English-Speaking Members Now Than English-Speaking.* Retrieved from https://www.lds.org/study/ensign/2000/09/news-of-the-church/historic-milestone-achieved-more-non-english-speaking-members-now-than-english-speaking?lang=eng.

Turcios-Cotto, V. Y., & Milan, S. (2013). Racial/ethnic differences in the educational expectations of adolescents: Does pursuing higher education mean something different to Latino students compared to White and Black students? *Journal of Youth and Adolescence, 42*(9), 1399–1412.

Weaver, S. J. (2018). *"Mormon" is out: Church releases statement on how to refer to the organization.* Retrieved from https://www.lds.org/church/news/mormon-is-out-church-releases-statement-on-how-to-refer-to-the-organization?lang=eng.

Chapter 6
Assumed Privilege and Role Confusion: A South Asian Woman's Experiences of Social Location and Professional Roles

Gita Seshadri

"Gen X and Millennial, South Asian, Female, Heterosexual, Spiritual, Acquired disability, Citizen, and non-indigenous"—Author's social locations. When I think of these words, I am often reminded of professional conferences. This may seem like an unnatural association; however, to me this is a direct reminder of when I am directly called to explore this work. Initially, exploring social location has been a more internal and self-examination process, however, writing this chapter has given me a bigger voice to examine more external processes related to my professional world. The intersections of my age, culture and ethnicity, gender, religion, and spirituality are frequently challenged by other dimensions of my identity with different metamessages (i.e., nonverbals and "shoulds" about labels)—for instance, my national origin (US citizen born to immigrant parents), educational background (university educated and in leadership positions), and generational influences (e.g., in between Generation X and Millennial)—give messages that are sometimes opposite of each other. This leaves me with a continual conundrum: Given that navigating these categories often requires me to exist in multiple worlds, both consciously and subconsciously, how do I honor many, if not all my social locations respectively? How does my intersectionality shape my experiences? Further, how do roles of authority, such as being a professor, clinician, or supervisor, influence these dynamics?

G. Seshadri (✉)
Couple and Family Therapy Program, Alliant International University, Sacramento, CA, USA
e-mail: gseshadri@alliant.edu

© Springer Nature Switzerland AG 2021
K. M.-T. Quek, A. L. Hsieh (eds.), *Intersectionality in Family Therapy Leadership*, AFTA SpringerBriefs in Family Therapy,
https://doi.org/10.1007/978-3-030-67977-4_6

Addressing Social Locations and Intersectionality

I will be using Hays' (2001) framework and compiling the ADDRESSING framework (i.e., age, disability, religion, ethnicity, socioeconomic status, sexual orientation, indigenous heritage, national origin, and gender) to explore these conundrums
through my own social cultural self-assessment and then use these applications to
delve into my educational roles.

Age

Although the Hays' 2001, 2008 and 2013 frameworks discuss age as a privileged
social location spanning from the ages of 18–65 (respectively) and lists minority
groups as children, adolescents, and elders, I do not agree with the author's thought
process that these ages are only considered markers of privilege; for me, I have
experienced it as an avenue of marginalization professionally. When others look at
me, I am often met with the feedback (subtly and indirectly or directly) that I carry
a very youthful appearance, so much so that early in my career and even now, I still
often receive questions and shaming comments, such as "How old are you? Your
voice sounds like you are 16!" and "How long have you been in the field?" To me
these questions and comments, though perhaps intending to be friendly, to me seem
to be a larger question of concerns around my competence and authority.

A small-scale example of this was during one of my classes in my first year as a
new full-time professor. I had made a reference to a then-25-year-old historical
event (i.e., the 1989 Loma Prieta earthquake) as a teaching point, and one student
(who identified as Caucasian, Christian, heterosexual, and male) stated at the end of
the lecture, "You were uncomfortably during that time?" and then quickly said,
"You don't have to answer that," and smiled. I responded affirmatively to answer his
question and showed a little surprise with a smile. Though the student caught the
microaggression referencing the implication of marginalization with his question,
(i.e., that I was too young to be a professor and/or that those who are professors
should be older), which was couched within his own privileged assumptions (i.e.,
that professors should be older), I could not help but wonder if this question would
have been raised if I had an older or otherwise different physical appearance, and
whether me being in a role of authority as a professor influenced the student's
assumptions about my age. Little did the student know that I was alive during the
earthquake, even though my students, including him, were not. In actuality, I had
been in the field for 10 years at that point. Hearing such comments made me feel
like I couldn't ignore that my knowledge and competence were being subtly ques-
tioned because of my apparent age, presumptions about what an authority figure
should look like, and/ or perhaps other intersections of my social locations that
make me who I am. Could it also be that deep down he was questioning me because
I am a person of color and female?

When most people think of discrimination in relation to age (i.e., ageism), it is usually in reference to older persons; in fact, even US law focuses its protections against age discrimination on individuals at or over the age of 40. Ageism is less commonly thought of as affecting those who are between the ages of 15 and 29 (Nadler, Morr, & Naumann, 2017). But emerging data show that Millennials feel discriminated against based on their age, experiencing this through microaggressions, generational stereotypes or stigma, and missed opportunities (Beaton, 2016; Bratt, Abrams, & Swift, 2020; Raymer, Reed, Spiegel, & Purvanova, 2017; Zabel et al., 2017). The literature also references this type of discrimination as reverse ageism. However, current US law offers no recourse for such discrimination, even though the consequences are real (Bratt et al., 2020), leaving those under the age of 40 unprotected. What is also relevant is that gender and racial and ethnic background were not emphasized as the focus of these studies. Based on this intersectionality, how would those factors influence?

In the next section, I will continue to explain how my culture, ethnicity, gender, and sexual orientation play a role in answering this presupposition within critical social theory (McDowell, 2015).

Culture, Ethnicity, Gender, and Sexual Orientation

I am a second-generation South Asian heterosexual female from a collectivist background. As the child of immigrants, I consider myself South Asian as well as American. This dual cultural identity means I sometimes receive conflicting instructions from my two cultures. For example, the implicit messages from my South Asian background regarding power and authority are to defer to elders and parents (because they deserve respect and have wisdom), men (because I am female), and those in authority (because I should be obedient); to marry young (between the ages of 20 and 29, to preserve naivety and social structure as a part of the patriarchy); and to not forget my culture. In contrast, the not-so-subtle messages from my American side are to be bold and assertive (because individualism is prized) but also assimilate to some degree to the dominant culture; to be educated and marry later in life; and to be direct (but not too direct, as I am female, and that would be impolite) (Bajaj, Natrajan-Tyagi, & Seshadri, 2016; Deepak, 2005; Natrajan-Tyagi, Seshadri, & Bajaj, 2016; Tuli, 2012).

Essentially, South Asian culture favors being in the background for the collective good, whereas American culture encourages being at the forefront with the goal of self-preservation. Even in the earthquake example, one could argue that my student's perception of me was influenced by not only my age, but also my ethnicity, as well as my gender. I believe this hidden conglomeration of assumptions impacts how others see me within my professional roles. For me, navigating the instructions from all of these contexts and social locations often gets confusing.

Although I do carry privilege on account of my heterosexual status, I still get questions from others (students, clients, and supervisees) about whether I am going to have an arranged marriage (influenced by their perceptions related to my ethnic background and race) due to their assumptions about my culture, presumptions about my age, and parental influences (deferring to elders), which are considered microaggressions. How does religion intersect in these dynamics?

Religion

I consider myself a spiritual person where I honor all religions and was raised with Hinduism. I still practice aspects of Hinduism and some Christian and American traditions (e.g., Christmas). Living in a country where Christianity is the dominant religion and having gone to a Christian university for graduate school (both masters and doctoral), I still have conflicting instructions on how to exist in these conflicting worlds. I have found that sometimes sharing that you are not part of the dominant discourse or privileged group regarding religion spurs behaviors from others that leave me feeling uncomfortable because their behavior highlights that I am different from them rather than the response showing the similarities between us or finding a bridge of commonality.

One client, after some investigation discovered that I did not belong to their religious group (Christianity) and decided to turn their treatment session into an opportunity to convert me to Christianity. Despite the client seeing me as being in the authority role as the therapist, the client felt it was necessary to make this a part of the treatment process. This moment felt oppressive because the client thought I needed to see the error of my ways instead of respecting my beliefs. Further, it did bother me that he turned his treatment into something other than what he was there for; however, I realized after the fact that this was a part of his avoidance. Perhaps, the client was also challenging other aspects of my minority identities too, including the perceived privilege of education.

Education and Ability

Being in the education sector and working at a university categorizes me as middle class and is inextricably linked to privilege. In addition, being a person of color (also darker skinned), I also serve as representation. Standing as the face of representation may even show other people of color that they can succeed in higher education and positions of authority previously reserved for the privileged elite. The fact that I had the option to pursue higher education is indicative of my privilege. However, it is worth noting the intersectionality of socioeconomic status; I did not have the privilege of funding my own education by paying out of pocket, which one might assume of someone from a higher social class. Like most students pursuing higher education, I had to secure student loans in the hopes that my earning potential would help take care of my debt, highlighting educational inequity (Krishnamoorthi & Kaissi, 2020).

More specifically, Tran, Mintert, Llamas, and Lam (2018) also discussed the implications of stress and debt for minority person's health during college, noting that Asians in the study experienced less stress than participants from other minority groups, perhaps due to seeing debt as a "necessary evil" tied to their educational pursuits (p. 465). In addition, the cost of education does not always translate into equity of what one is paid with a salary upon graduation. This gap is also influenced by age, gender, and race and ethnicity. Most importantly, while education is a privilege, the literal added price tag of carrying debt and the metaphorical price tag of paying off debt contribute to my mixed experiences regarding the privilege associated with education.

Ability status, though invisible, also plays a role in my identity and social locations. I have had a chronic health issue (i.e., food allergies /sensitivities) that is a nonvisible disability that has affected my adult life. It often requires that I have special accommodations and is not itself a source of privilege. To others, this may result in the appearance of privilege because of my self-advocacy around it (e.g., asking for special menus and modifications, requesting specific restaurants, etc.), and it requires me to be assertive and request accommodations, a behavior that clashes with my other social locations and may appear to others as snobby or bourgeois. In the past, others have disagreed with my advocacy for myself because it appears to them (based on their assumptions and discomfort) that I am requesting accommodations based on my preferences and pickiness rather than as a need for survival and quality of life. I have also had some try to metaphorically or literally control my plate by saying "you shouldn't be eating this or that" based on their own knowledge on the subject. Professionally, this can show up when clients desire to give me gifts, when students and colleagues express a desire to have potlucks, and when I and my supervisees need to have "working lunches or dinners" and eat during meetings. As you can see, these situations are not clear; needing to be a chameleon while sometimes feeling like I am performing magic acts because I exist in multiple worlds is key here. This also influences my roles in the mental health field.

Privilege in Mental Health

My professional roles of clinician, supervisor, and professor are automatically tagged with power and privilege; various social constructs attribute meaning related to authority and expertise to these positions based on their titles alone. However, exploring my intersectionality mandates that I also evaluate the social instructions of these roles as well. It is difficult to say that only one of the social categories experienced is the whole experience or can be experienced in isolation (McDowell, 2015).

When I think about my visible identity, I imagine only a few of my social locations being recognized immediately based on visible differences (e.g., gender and ethnicity). It may take a little bit longer for others to accurately identify my socioeconomic status, education level, and age, and may presuppose at first glance. In considering how my readily visible traits compare to my self-identification via social locations, I feel these traits do not fully represent my experiences and can trigger automatic assumptions of assumed privilege from others. The constellation of my social locations also influences how others see me. Professionally, being a South Asian female also plays a role. My perception is that youth may be valued in society as a whole; however, in the mental health profession, because one is seen as an authority regardless of capacity (e.g., clinician, supervisor, professor/leader), wisdom, seniority, and age-related experiences take precedence. Also, most founders of family therapy theories were upper class, Caucasian, Christian, and abled men, who were citizens. Being a woman of color with a youthful appearance unquestionably plays a part in my professional roles.

The issue of visibility and invisibility in the professional context may often refer to self-disclosure and projection (Chalfin, 2014). There is little research on self-disclosure and projection as applied to ethnic minority therapists; most studies have been done with therapists of the majority culture (Fong, 2016). However, Fong (2016, abstract) discusses that the issue of "… race and ethnicity becomes one of power and privilege, oppression, and subjugation. This process can be crude, often evoking a deep human vulnerability within the minority clinician." Further, Fong (2016) adds, this process is a part of the therapeutic relationship and must be continually negotiated with the client.

Being a Clinician

Working in mental health most often puts clinicians in a privileged position, as the authority figure in the role of helping clients changes their lives. Integrating my social locations and identity as well as power can create a sense of awkwardness because I can simultaneously inhabit both disadvantaged and privileged roles during the therapeutic dance. In this section, I will discuss the nuances of this, including how therapeutic practices coupled with my social locations/identity can intersect (i.e., age/authority, education/wealth, ability/health, and heritage/ambiguity).

I believe that being female and heterosexual contributes to clients seeing me as nurturing and warm. Some have coupled this with my ethnic origin to view me as more traditional; others seem to see it as a form of connection. Though I see myself as a guide, clients often come to therapy seeking advice and formal direction. This power differential can show up in the beginning of the therapeutic relationship. Questions about why I am in the field, what my story is, and why did I decide to become a therapist are various questions that I receive. I perceive this as my clients' way of making a deeper inquiry around my related experiences: "Can and do you understand me? Are you able to help me? Can you understand my life experiences?" I try to respond empathically to this question and explore clients' perspectives regarding what is blocking them from reaching their goals.

Some clients also pose another question, either subtly or in more direct ways: "What have you been through that proves to me that you can relate to me?" I see their questions and behavior as a reflection of their perceived assumptions about my being a person of color and female. For example, these questions show up out of a natural desire on the clients' part to connect based on perceived similarities and later may disappear if clients are able to work past their perceptions and assumptions about their therapists. Usually, this is done after they establish a therapeutic connection and relationship with their therapist through feeling vulnerability (Nienhuis et al., 2018).

Yet, clients likely assume I am more privileged than I am, due to their assumptions about me or what I represent. I believe that this may be a result of the privilege I carry on account of my profession and the titles that I have earned. For example, mandated clients have assumed my privilege is connected to being a part of the system that they are fighting against, and/or other clients have assumed that being university educated means I am wealthy. Relatedly, my chronic health issue is often invisible until I bring attention to it (this is extremely rare, due to it not being relevant in session). For example, when a client offers me food (as a gift), it can create an additional level of discomfort due to not only having to explain policies around therapists accepting gifts, but also briefly explaining my chronic health issue, and perhaps the client feeling pressure to accommodate me. For me, having to do so brings conversations challenging assumptions, projection, and/or self-disclosure.

Regarding whether to accept gifts from clients, some practitioners are more inclined to abide by a rigid guideline of not accepting gifts, whereas the decision is less clear for others. The need to responsibly work within this complexity challenges many of my other social locations, which can reinforce privilege. For example, I tend to be a more cautious person, which appears to stem from my South Asian values (being in the background), but it also highlights the assumption of my American values—the expectation that clients should be more understanding about this because it is associated with the profession. I reflect constantly on these kinds of tensions as I try to determine what is appropriate or fair to the client.

In addition, my university education is an indicator of my privilege. This influences the way that I talk, think, how I was trained, and adds to my aura of being an old soul. Coupled with my youthful appearance, I think this may confuse clients and sometimes even students as well. To bridge this, I tell clients and students that they do not have to address me as "Doctor," and I often introduce myself with my first name. To me, my titles do not matter; I care more about having respectful relationships in which both parties contribute. This is my way of trying to equalize power as well as demonstrate that I do not try to live in a metaphoric ivory tower, where I am too far removed from their experiences because of my university education, supervisory, and professorial roles. I try to put myself in my clients' shoes and even try to imagine how I would feel if I were living their lives. While recognizing the merit and respect of my positions and still desiring more equal relationships with clients and students, this also can sometimes produce a tension within myself and sometimes with a client when I am using the lenses of family therapy theorist founders that I have been taught (e.g., theory), as the theories have been primarily developed through avenues of privilege and traditionally practiced with clients of majority backgrounds.

I am also not of indigenous heritage. However, throughout my life others have confused my ethnic identity due to ambiguity regarding racial and ethnic categorizations—which could be described as Indian, South Asian, or East Indian—with the Native American Indian background; the conflating of identities tends to happen to persons inhabiting multiple minority groups (Aspinall, 2002). Further, others also make assumptions about my national origin as evidenced by questions about where I am from. The continuous conundrum presents itself in the way I wish to go about it—desiring to share what is relevant, beneficial to the client, therapeutically appropriate, change inducing (if necessary) and connecting. I find that this is also moderated by my therapeutic relationship with my client.

I think that in group settings with clients, I use a similar approach yet tend to share less about myself in alignment with practice due to group dynamics that are naturally present. I also tend to share less when I feel assumptions are placed on me, whether in one-on-one or group interactions, due to not initially feeling a sense of safety. My solution to the question above is that I tend to process those interactions emotional with clients by trying to understand where their assumed belief around assumed privilege is coming from even though I seem to be the immediate catalyst, or if it is in fact related to me directly. And, when I am not in the presence of the client, I self-reflect regarding my own countertransference or use anonymous consult.

Being a Supervisor

I am a supervisor of supervisees, and I also supervise supervisors through the AAMFT supervision certification. I see the relationship between myself, other supervisors, and my supervisees as a collaborative, despite the intentional hierarchy and power dynamics that the titles bring. The intersections of my social locations, my supervisees' and supervisors' locations need to be evaluated in a parallel way. I often ask supervisees and supervisors to talk about their social locations in relation to their clients when they are doing case presentations or, in the case of supervisors, talking about their supervisees. By having this as a part of the discussion, there is a dialogue regarding the multiple systems at work. Reflecting upon this, I also notice that I tend to have stronger boundaries around self-disclosure with clients than with supervisees or supervisors; despite all of these relationships being collaborative, I use more caution with clients due to a desire to create an environment, where the client can focus on themselves. Speaking about social locations with my supervisees or supervisors also seems to come more naturally to me due to associating this with my university education, class discussions, and consultations.

With supervisees and supervisors, I share my social locations as they may apply to the case and shape how the supervisee can have a discussion with their client regarding the client's presenting problem, themselves, and myself as the supervisor.

Talking about how these social locations and how they relate to the presenting issues helps me contextualize to understand what my supervisees and supervisors are struggling with. It also helps to identify my own countertransference and biases.

I see the intersectionality of almost all my social locations, including age, being a female of color, being in the position of authority, university educated, spiritual, and not being of indigenous heritage, and ability as part of what supervisees and supervisors may challenge when there are problems in the supervisory relationship. For example, when training a female supervisor who was older than me, the elephant in the room became difficulties around receiving guidance from me due to the fact that she perceived me as significantly younger than her and would display this in her offhand comments, yet having to receive feedback due to the nature of our relationship.

As discussed in the clinician section, privilege can show up when adhering to professional standards; the same applies here. I see it in the implied hierarchy of the supervisor-supervisee relationship and between supervisors and myself, a supervisor of supervisors. For example, my recommendations could be translated as an implied "You must do..." mandate rather than an inquiry along the lines of "What do you think about trying this?" To share identities and social locations within multiple worlds, I try to engage each supervisor in conversation about power dynamics with the client or supervisee, as well as our relationship. If the supervisor, supervisee, or client does not bring up issues of privilege and social oppression, I feel it is my responsibility to have these conversations with them. By engaging in these processes in this manner, jumping between multiple worlds feels more natural.

Being a Professor/Leader

There are many levels of privilege in the classroom. Assumed privilege lies with the person in the role of professor, as this is someone in authority providing instruction to students. Assumed privilege is important to explore in that it highlights perception around social location and refers to projection and intersectionality. I have noticed that since I became tenured, I feel more comfortable sharing about myself, whereas before I was more hesitant. Tobin (2010) also references this process in exploring self-disclosure in teaching. The author cites Michelle Payne's commentary of women in authority in a similar way to Rahimi and Askari Bigdeli's (2016) discussion on outside factors:

> Michelle Payne offers a compelling personal narrative that suggests how and why it could be riskier for a young, female, relatively inexperienced instructor to preach and practice a pedagogy of decentered authority than it would be for an instructor who is older, male, and tenured. I'd suggest that the same is true with regard to self-disclosure. In other words, adopting a controversial political position or telling a story about some personal failure is likely to pose very different risks for different teachers working in different contexts (pp. 200–201).

Based on this, I realized that being female and of South Asian descent (i.e., a double minority), I felt that students would take a more critical view of me, which is supported by the above references. When students perceive a younger female of minority status and other quality differences, they tend to be more critical (Payne, 1994; Rahimi & Askari Bigdeli, 2016). I experienced this when teaching a diversity course. In students' course evaluation and feedback, there were subtle requests for me to be clearer in my communication as well as more direct feedback around how I pronounced words and my word choice to describe certain concepts. Relatedly, research also shows that students tend to be critical when they perceive their professor as different than them (Rahimi & Askari Bigdeli, 2016; Simpson, 2009). I would argue that this can run across all my social locations because the intersection produces a minority identity on multiple levels. The students' implied message in this scenario is often "I know better than you and you should do it this way." These processes highlight intersectionality around multiple social locations and assumed privilege.

By default, what is invisible to me in the classroom are certain aspects of the ADDRESSING values that students do not share initially beyond what is visible (e.g., new students who have yet to share their experiences or those who are more introverted or shy and choose to keep the information more to themselves). This can make the situation feel like we are all in a magic act, not knowing how to respond to the societal audience because everyone is taking in the environment, and the invisible (i.e., students' unshared social locations) has yet to be made visible.

Being a faculty of color (i.e., a faculty member of minority status by race, culture, and/or ethnicity), I see what is discussed in the classroom around these values, but I also have my own intuitions about what my students are thinking. Admittedly, I do have high expectations of my students because I believe they can succeed. I try to equalize barriers based on the conversations that I have with my students around social location, but after becoming tenured, I am more intentional of setting the tone of the classroom to ensure a certain level of emotional safety so that students will be more willing to share, and I in turn share as well. I also understand that for a person of color, judgment is experienced differently than of someone who has more levels of privilege; it's harder for a person who has less privileges to confront judgment due to their limited physical and emotional resources.

Students respond to me based on their projections, regarding my social identities and power contexts. This might be apparent in students' questions, comments, or observations they make about me. Many times, students keep their actual perceptions to themselves, and I sometimes only see these come out when they complete evaluations, whether they be formal or informal. This is at times frustrating for me, but I can also see how my assumed role of authority and privilege can be a barrier in this regard. On the opposite side of the coin, sometimes students tend to gravitate toward me because of their knowledge of my academic and clinical expertise. Other times, I wonder if it is because they feel that I am more in alignment with their social locations, or perhaps they feel connected to me based on some limited self-disclosure. Most likely, all can be true.

Lastly, my communication style is influenced by my social location and the metamessages I have received that students would prefer I be more direct. This could be due to them wanting me to rely more on my American values, or it could be the manifestation of a disconnect between reality and their expectations. For example, I get questions regarding assignments that essentially ask, "What are you looking for?" I include rubrics and explain assignments in class, including highlighting which sections might require or emphasize creativity. But I still receive anxiously based questions from students who want more clarity. One might chalk this up to a generational difference—that is, students want me to tell them how to do it, as opposed to trying something on their own with the risk of it not being what is asked of them—or trying to find a cookie-cutter way of completing the assignment. Sometimes I feel confused about what exactly they are asking for and why.

Conclusion

Intersectionality deserves in-depth analysis; a simple checking of the box in an assessment does not do it justice. Through this discussion of my social locations and the ways they play out in my personal and professional capacities, I noticed that my own parallel process was to recognize on a deeper level the importance of exploring the ADDRESSING values in many capacities within the privileged world of mental health. This is a reciprocal process that requires having multiple and constant conversations about social locations. I appreciate the opportunity to undertake the exploration of social intersectionality in my professional life; to not undertake this work would make the invisible even more hidden and the unavoidable creation of more performances of magic acts. I feel that undertaking this work, as it relates to me during my journey of life, puts me on a course of making humble, thoughtful, and considered decisions about my responses to others, and more reflective of others' responses to me, and therefore, makes me more confident and less anxious about the nature and quality of my professional path.

Acknowledgments I would like to thank my colleagues (Drs. Alex Hsieh, Karen Quek, and the other authors of this text) for providing the opportunity to engage in this work at a deeper and academic level. I would also like to thank Dr. Carmen Knudson-Martin for her edits and mentoring, and Dr. Naveen Johnathan for our continual collegial conversations throughout our careers that pushed me to get to the heart of my voice within all my identities and reconcile what it means to be both South Asian and American for each of us over the years. Also, I would like to thank my parents who have raised me to have analytical mind, and Patrick, my significant other, who emotionally supports me and kept me on my toes with interesting and engaging debates about social location and intersectionality nuances as I wrote this chapter. And finally, I would like to thank my clients, students/supervisees, and supervisors for helping to plant seeds of curiosity along my journey and a desire to do this work in honor of them and myself.

References

Aspinall, P. J. (2002). Collective terminology to describe the minority ethnic population: The persistence of confusion and ambiguity in usage. *Sociology, 36*(4), 803–816. https://doi.org/10.1177/0038038502036000401.

Bajaj, A. A., Natrajan-Tyagi, R., & Seshadri, G. (2016, July). *Communication Patterns in Indian American Immigrant Families: A workshop for future generations.* Workshop presented at the first annual South Asian Mental Health conference, Union City, CA.

Beaton, C. (2016, November 11). Too young to lead? When youth works against you. *Forbes.* Retrieved from: https://www.forbes.com/sites/carolinebeaton/2016/11/11/too-young-to-lead-when-youth-works-against-you/#4a85067f3c2a.

Bratt, C., Abrams, D., & Swift, H. J. (2020). Supporting the old but neglecting the young? The two faces of ageism. *Developmental Psychology, 56*(5), 1029–1039. https://doi.org/10.1037/dev0000903. (Supplemental).

Chalfin. (2014). The role of a visible/visual disability in the clinical dyad: Issues of visibility/invisibility for the client and clinician. *Psychoanalytic Social Work, 21*(1–2), 121–132. https://doi.org/10.1080/15228878.2013.834265.

Deepak, A. C. (2005). Parenting and the process of migration: Possibilities within south Asian families. *Child Welfare League of America, 84*, 585–606.

Fong, T. (2016). The ambiguous other: Reflections on race and culture in the assessment relationship. In B. L. Mercer, T. Fong, & E. Rosenblatt (Eds.), *Assessing children in the urban community* (pp. 89–95). New York, NY: Routledge/Taylor & Francis Group.

Hays, P. A. (2001). *Addressing cultural complexities in practice: A framework for clinicians and counselors.* Washington, DC: American Psychological Association.

Hays, P. A. (2008). *Addressing cultural complexities in practice: Assessment, diagnosis, and therapy* (2nd ed.). Washington, DC: American Psychological Association.

Hays, P. A. (2013). *Connecting across cultures: The Helper's toolkit* (pp. 15–16). Thousand Oaks, CA: SAGE. Original version published in Hays, P. A. (2008). *Addressing cultural complexities in practice: Assessment, diagnosis, and therapy.* Washington DC: APA. Retrieved from https://division45.org/wp-content/uploads/2015/06/CulturalPsychology.pdf.

Krishnamoorthi, R., & Kaissi, B. (2020). The college transparency act: Strengthening transparency, equity, and student success in American higher education. *Harvard Journal on Legislation, 57*(1), 1–23.

McDowell, T. (2015). *Applying critical social theories to family therapy practice.* Cham, Switzerland: Springer International Publishing. https://doi.org/10.1007/978-3-319-15633-0.

Nadler, J. T., Morr, R., & Naumann, S. (2017). Millennials, media, and research: Ageism and the younger worker. In E. Parry & J. McCarthy (Eds.), *The Palgrave handbook of age diversity and work* (pp. 423–446). London, UK: Palgrave. https://doi.org/10.1057/978-1-137-46781-2.

Natrajan-Tyagi, R., Seshadri, G., & Bajaj, A. A. (2016, February). *Communication patterns in Indian American immigrant families: A workshop for future generations.* Workshop presented at the sixth annual AAMFT-CA conference, San Francisco, CA.

Nienhuis, J. B., Owen, J., Valentine, J. C., Winkeljohn Black, S., Halford, T. C., Parazak, S. E., et al. (2018). Therapeutic alliance, empathy, and genuineness in individual adult psychotherapy: A meta-analytic review. *Psychotherapy Research, 28*(4), 593–605. https://doi.org/10.1080/10503307.2016.1204023.

Payne, M. L. Tobin & T. Newkirk (Eds.) *Rendering women's authority in the writing classroom. Taking stock: The writing process movement in the 90s* (Vol. 1994, pp. 97–111). Portsmouth: Boynton/Cook.

Rahimi, A., & Askari Bigdeli, R. (2016). Iranian EFL teachers' perceptions of teacher self-disclosure. *Iranian Journal of Language Teaching Research, 4*(1), 83–96.

Raymer, M., Reed, M., Spiegel, M., & Purvanova, R. K. (2017). An examination of generational stereotypes as a path towards reverse ageism. *The Psychologist-Manager Journal, 20*(3), 148–175. https://doi.org/10.1037/mgr0000057.

Simpson, K. (2009). Did I just share too much information? Results of a national survey on faculty self-disclosure. *International Journal of Teaching and Learning in Higher Education, 20*(2), 91–97.

Tobin, L. (2010). OPINION: Self-disclosure as a strategic teaching tool: What I do and don't tell my students. *College English, 73*(2), 196–206.

Tran, A. G. T. T., Mintert, J. S., Llamas, J. D., & Lam, C. K. (2018). At what costs? Student loan debt, debt stress, and racially/ethnically diverse college students' perceived health. *Cultural Diversity & Ethnic Minority Psychology, 24*(4), 459–469. https://doi.org/10.1037/cdp0000207.

Tuli, M. (2012). Beliefs on parenting and childhood in India. *Journal of Comparative Family Studies, 43*(1), 81–91.

Zabel, K. L., Biermeier-Hanson, B. B. J., Baltes, B. B., Early, B. J., & Shepard, A. (2017). Generational differences in work ethic: Fact or fiction? *Journal of Business and Psychology, 32*(3), 301–315. https://doi.org/10.1007/s10869-016-9466-5.

Chapter 7
Story of a Taiwanese Female Postmodern MFT Faculty: Supervisory Practices in a Cross-Cultural Context

Hao-Min Chen

The multiple environments I have lived in and experienced shape my story as a postmodern supervisor. In this chapter, I begin with a narrative about my family of origin, cross-cultural life journey, and the social location in which I have been immersed; this narrative leads to the story of why I chose to adopt postmodern approaches in my work, and how I perceive myself applying postmodern supervision in MFT practicum classes in the USA. My identity as a Taiwanese female faculty member adds multiple layers of complexity to this account, as these intersectional experiences influence my understanding and practice of postmodern supervision.

How Did I Get Here?

I was born and raised in Taiwan. My first language is Mandarin-Chinese. My parents were traditional middle-class Taiwanese who valued education, hard work, and perseverance. My dad was a faculty member at a university and the family's main bread earner. He was considered "higher social class" compared to my mom because of his graduate degree and occupation. My mom, like many Taiwanese women at that time, did not finish college and stayed at home to take care of her family (Lee & Mock, 2005a). Despite numerous conflicts in their relationship, my parents remained married for 38 years until my mom passed away a few years ago. In my memories, my mom submitted to my dad most of the time despite her short temper and seemly strong and, at times, overbearing personality.

H.-M. Chen (✉)
Marriage and Family Therapy Program, Texas A & M University-Central Texas, Killeen, TX, USA
e-mail: hmchen@tamuct.edu

© Springer Nature Switzerland AG 2021
K. M.-T. Quek, A. L. Hsieh (eds.), *Intersectionality in Family Therapy Leadership*, AFTA SpringerBriefs in Family Therapy,
https://doi.org/10.1007/978-3-030-67977-4_7

My parents' marriage seemed traditional and patriarchal in terms of gender roles, finances, and power. As a traditional ciswoman, my mom was subservient to my dad in many aspects of life (Ashton & Jordal, 2019). She was also expected to take full responsibility for the emotional support and domestic care of the family (Quek, Knudson-Martin, Orpen, & Victor, 2011). Growing up, I witnessed how dominant discourses of traditional and patriarchal cultural values, such as gender roles, governed the ways my parents thought of themselves, interacted with each other, and made meaning of their personal and family life (Walsh, 2019).

When I was little, my mom tried tirelessly but still struggled to meet the traditional Taiwanese cultural expectations placed on her—the foremost of which was to give birth to a son. As Lee and Mock (2005a) described, the value of a wife in Chinese culture was judged by her ability to produce a male heir. Sons were often favored more than daughters and were expected to carry on the family's name and legacy and to take care of their elderly parents (Hsieh & Bean, 2014). Daughters, on the other hand, were to be seen in relation to the men in their families, such as their fathers, husbands, and sons. Influenced by this traditional cultural and gender belief, my mom endured multiple doctor visits and medical consultations for infertility and alternative surgeries. She often took me with her to those appointments for company and emotional support. Sadly, after years of unsuccessful attempts, she gradually realized that she would never have a biological son of her own. She was met with the cruel disappointment that she had failed the predominant cultural expectation for a wife and could not have "a son to rely on" when she was old. She also treated my aunts who had sons with jealousy and envy and showed favoritism to my male cousins as if they were hers. She never said any demeaning things to me directly about my gender, but I remember those moments that I was puzzled and hurt by her obvious favoritism toward my male cousins.

As realistic and resilient as she was, my mom struggled to accept her situation, and eventually came to terms with it over time. She gradually unpacked her gender role stories within her social contexts, cultural surroundings, and life trajectory. During this reflection process, she found her own way to fight back against her gender fate as well as the male-centered culture (Ashton & Jordal, 2019). She spoke of sacrificing her education and career development opportunities to take care of her immediate and extended family; as a consequence, she lacked necessary knowledge and skills to find a well-paying job and had to be financially dependent on her husband. Her possibilities were constrained, and her choices within relationships were limited. For example, she had no choice but to take on the full responsibility of household chores. She suffered from the negative influence of the dominant gender discourse in her life that a woman had to be relationship-focused and was the assumed caregiver of the family. Thus, she demanded that I pursue higher education, get a professional job, and "never have to rely on men." She was determined to raise me like a son in her mind—a person who is well-educated, motivated, and career-driven; a professional who is financially independent and she can rely on when she is old.

My parents seldom agreed on things, but they both valued my education. They prized upward mobility and placed great importance on hard work and academic achievements. In this traditional Taiwanese belief system, ones' education level, career attainment, and work role contributed momentously to their self-esteem and self-definition (Lee & Mock, 2005b). Parents' childrearing practice and the face of the family could depend on the children's school performance as well as their future career achievements. Researchers have found that many Chinese immigrant parents bring this value from their country of origin to the USA (Hsieh & Bean, 2014).

Under the influence of this dominant cultural storyline and my mom's determination for me to pursue higher education, my parents invested a great portion of their time, money, and resources in my education. Even though they were not affluent, I was sent to numerous after-school programs on varied topics, such as science, math, language, art, and calligraphy. My mom would always wait patiently outside the classroom and talk with the teachers afterward regarding my overall progress in the particular subject. My room was filled with educational materials, including audiobooks, classic works of literature, children's encyclopedias, and science kits. For more than 12 years, a hired tutor would come to my home to give me weekly or biweekly private piano lessons. It was not until my first year in college that my mom finally gave up on me ever becoming the pianist she wanted me to be. I still remember the distress, disappointment, passive-aggressiveness, and bitterness in her voice when she said, "You don't have to play if you don't like it. It's just a waste of money."

During vacation breaks, my mom loved to travel and often brought me along. We visited many countries in Europe, North America, and different parts of Asia. She carefully selected trips with guided tours and live commentaries so that I could learn more about the local history, customs, and traditions. She insisted that these trips had to be both fun and educational and, at the end of the day, asked questions to test me on what I had learned from the attractions and sightseeing. I occasionally would throw a temper tantrum because of these annoying "quizzes" but was often quickly distracted by all the interesting and exciting things happening around me overseas.

Although I enjoyed the varied learning experiences, consistent with Lee and Mock's (2005a) cultural observation of some Chinese mothers, I felt my mom was somewhat overbearing, guilt-inducing, and overinvolved with my life. Growing up, I had a love-hate relationship with her and had always felt some level of stress and anxiety about my performance. In Taiwan, this academic stress and pressure from parents to succeed seemed fairly common, and was considered the norm; researchers, however, have found it to correlate with adolescent depression (Gao et al., 2020). The pressure to succeed was also associated with high levels of stress, academic anxiety, somatic complaints, and shame upon oneself and the entire family for Asian American individuals (Hsieh & Bean, 2014).

However, looking back through a postmodern perspective that understands a person from her own context, my mom might just have been doing what she knew best in raising me. She was determined to push me to be different (from the traditional image of a Taiwanese woman/wife) and not "repeat the same mistakes I made in my life." Her seemingly controlling demeanor within the parent-child relationship was a reflection of her conformity and suffering and, eventually, a carefully considered response to the socially constructed expectations imposed by the larger cultural aggregation and people around her. As Walsh (2019) stated, "Our lives exist and take on meaning within the social worlds that have shaped us and through which we negotiate our path in life" (p. 49).

In addition, though I had mixed feelings about my mom's and the Taiwanese academic and career expectations, I was privileged in terms of my educational opportunities and resources. The after-school programs, private lessons, and international travel experiences had not only equipped me with specific academic knowledge and skills to compete with my peers in school but also had given me access to a wider range of sociocultural narratives and life choices (Freedman and Combs, 1996). This background knowledge as well as the formal and informal ways of learning prepared me well to seek higher education in Taiwan and in the USA, which, later on, helped me find a professional job and a satisfying career. These initial encounters with diverse cultures, worldviews, and realities during traveling promoted my current interests as well as my understanding of postmodern theories.

After finishing my bachelor's degree at the best university in Taiwan, I pursued my "American dream" and obtained my master's and doctoral degrees in marriage and family therapy (MFT) in the USA. My mom did not know this major well but was proud of my degrees. Since then, I have been in the field of MFT for almost two decades—starting as an adjunct instructor and clinical supervisor in the USA and Taiwan, and eventually took on a core faculty in MFT programs in the USA. My mom was instrumental in my career advancement. Like many women in collective cultures, she viewed my achievements as her own success (Lee & Mock, 2005b). Because of her sacrifice and perseverance, I was able to build my career, maintain a professional job, and be financially independent in my marriage. My accomplishments, which she had planned and worked hard for, led to changes in certain aspects of my default gender role and contributed to a more equal relationship between my husband and me, compared to my parents. My situation reflects Quek and Knudson-Martin's (2008) research, which explored wives' paid employment, educational attainment, and the sense of control they had over their own lives played an important role in gender equality in marriage. This did not necessarily mean that spouses fully shared power in every other aspect of their relationship. Nevertheless, acknowledging wives as coproviders in the family created changes in the arrangement of implicit but influential household tasks as well as related decision processes. For example, these husbands may initiate more household responsibilities, actively recognize and value their wives' contributions, and willingly share mutual prioritization of wives' careers (Quek et al., 2011).

From an individualist mainstream point of view, my mom might still be viewed as "a housewife with no professional skills or further career development." However, in traditional Taiwanese culture, which emphasizes interdependence more than independence, my academic and career achievements were considered a collective effort and a success shared by me, her, and the family. As the main caregiver, she deserved the credit and had the right to brag about it with friends and relatives. She saved face, and her contribution was recognized and celebrated. She also proved that it is not impossible to change one's gender fate of having to be financially dependent on men (e.g., our husbands and sons), and a daughter could bring her and the family honor not only through the man she marries, but also through her own educational and career achievement. In a collective way, my mom reclaimed the disavowed parts of herself that had struggled to survive under the constraint of dominant discourse, patriarchy, and other structures of marginalization (Ashton & Jordal, 2019). Her feelings that her possibilities were constrained and her space was limited by the gender roles and traditional cultural beliefs were somewhat alleviated.

My relationship with my mom shaped my beliefs and perspectives about culture, gender role, and marriage, which planted a seed for my future learning and practice of the postmodern perspective. However, at that time, I was not able to identify those transformative life experiences or articulate those underlying emotional and thinking processes. It was only after learning the systemic theory and postmodern approach that I was able to further process and integrate my relationship with my mom as I put all the broken pieces together—the strong influences of the social norms and taken-for-granted assumptions, the mainstream narratives, our social locations and associated privileges and subjugations, as well as how one's personal agency and resiliency in life could create a unique outcome for me and my family.

Different Systems, Different Expectations

My husband and I met in the USA while I was attending graduate school. We are both Taiwanese and share the value of the cultural emphasis on education and career achievement of many Asian immigrant families (Hsieh & Bean, 2014). As a joint decision, we moved several times internationally and across different states to pursue the best educational and career opportunities for each or both of us. Many times, we moved to a location far from relatives and friends, spent a couple of years making it home, and moved again shortly thereafter. Looking back, there is a Chinese saying that perfectly describes our bold decision process—初生之犢不畏虎— which literally translates as "the newborn calf is not afraid of tigers." Relocating without much social support and rebuilding a personal network from scratch was time-consuming and emotionally draining, but I was too young, and perhaps too entitled, to realize it.

Moving internationally from Taiwan to the USA for graduate school was not easy. It was a major shift in my social and power context—I was transformed from a middle-class college graduate to a "fresh off the boat" foreigner who did not know much about her surroundings. The visible and hidden agendas in my new environment demanded an utterly different skillset. Despite being motivated and career-driven, I was trained well according to the more traditional aspects of Taiwanese culture, which values being quiet, respectful, and considerate, focusing on others' needs more than yours, sacrificing without complaint, and tolerating people's mistakes instead of raising concerns. However, in the USA, these characteristics may be seen as lacking clear and effective communication, assertiveness, leadership, and healthy interpersonal boundaries. It took me several years to realize this, create my own technical definitions of "cultural differences," and learn basic survival skills for the USA.

In the classroom, there were many times when I was the only non-native English speaker. Although I had qualified education, training, and professional experiences, grammar mistakes in my speaking and oral presentations would easily undermine my credibility as a competent clinician and instructor. I was not able to sound precise, convincing, and persuasive—qualities that characterize the speech of typical authority figures in the dominant US culture and which a student might expect. In the early years of my teaching career, I received negative feedback in teaching evaluations relating to this issue. Although I provided many written materials (e.g., syllabus, PowerPoint slides, and grading rubrics), some students indicated that they felt my verbal instructions were confusing and inconsistent and claimed this was the main reason why they failed an assignment or exam; notably, others in the class were able to complete these tasks satisfactorily. Some students asked the same questions again and again in an attempt to elicit a different answer and find an easy way out. As a female faculty member of color, I seem to be more vulnerable to receiving this kind of criticism, and the students could perceive me as having less authority, righteousness, and credibility to begin with.

My "passive" and "vague" communication style was not only an issue of English speaking skills, but also a practiced cultural custom. Compared to traditional Taiwanese culture, American culture is relatively low-context and relies more on direct and explicit verbal communication. Information and rules in the USA are expected to be clearly spelled out and communicated primarily through language. On the other hand, traditional Taiwanese culture is high-context, which means it focuses on the interpersonal relationship and the implied messages within a specific group or context when communicating. Nonverbal behaviors and the group's identification and understanding, instead of direct language, are emphasized (Sue & Sue, 2012). The American cultural emphasis on verbal communication was embedded in the teaching evaluation; consequently, the evaluation could disadvantage an international faculty member like me whose original culture is relatively high-context and whose first language is not English. My experience is hardly unique: Fan et al. (2019) observed that teachers from non-English speaking backgrounds generally receive lower ratings compared to their native English-speaker counterparts.

Despite experiencing many scenarios in which I felt marginalized, I have been blessed with many kind, sincere, and honest people in my life, including compassionate mentors, caring supervisors and senior administration, friendly colleagues, generous acquaintances, and considerate students, all from various cultures. They have respected me and have created space for me as a minority female faculty member. I am deeply appreciative of their inclusivity. This mix of positive, negative, marginalized, and empowering experiences helped me to improve in my academic role and to apprehend the nuances of the influences of social location, particularly its effect on teaching and supervisory relationships.

Not One Way or the Other

The postmodern approach helped me understand the students and myself as a person and as a supervisor within various social and cultural contexts. For instance, from this perspective, the negative comments in my previous teaching evaluation were not judgments of each other as ignorant students or an incompetent instructor, but rather could be viewed as more of a mismatch of expectations instead of accusations or blame. Some students might have compared me with an inner image of an authority figure that looks, sounds, and behaves like the mainstream and meets the cultural emphasis on high verbal communication. This assumption was created by the dominant discourse and social settings as well as their previous interpersonal relationships. Likewise, I acted and responded based on my own cultural beliefs and what I thought was "right." However, looking through the postmodern lens, no one was necessarily "right" or "wrong." The students and I were in parallel universes that did not understand or connect with each other. As the theory suggests, perceptions and emotions, which are often considered to generate solely within the individual, are, in fact, influenced by the environment (Crotty, 1998). Judgments and evaluations that seemed personal were actually socially constructed. The so-called "truths" are shaped by cultural contexts and are intersubjective.

In other words, my students and I as their supervisor are not able to be objective and "bias-free." As Anderson (1997) stated, "A therapist cannot be neutral. All are impossible. On the contrary, we each take who we are, and all that that entails—personal and professional life experiences, values, biases, and convictions-with us into the therapy room" (p. 137). We all are "biased." We are biased because we understand the world based on our experiences of family of origin, gender, sexual orientation, ethnic identity, socioeconomic status, education, etc.

This postmodern perspective provided a justification for my differences—my quietness, lacking clear boundaries, passive and vague communication style, and etc. It gave me some space and a reason not to be fully "Americanized," as no culture or individual is "higher" or "better" than the other. We are just different, biased in our own way with our unique strengths and weakness. It allowed me to be myself and not lose my culture. At the same time, I was able to acknowledge, respect, support, and work with the various realities and expectations of my students and the overall western academic culture. This acknowledgment of different possibilities of being and interacting helped me to not hold grudges when receiving criticism, either constructive or sometimes, unfortunately, malicious. I learned to see the judgments from others as socially, culturally, and family constructed, instead of a purely personal attack. This viewpoint encouraged and consoled me when experiencing interpersonal conflicts and feeling marginalized as a faculty member of color. It helped me to keep an overall positive attitude and to see the persons and their real needs beyond their defenses. Postmodernism also addressed the power differences within the social context of academia, which shed light on the confusions around the power issues that I faced every day as a female faculty of color.

Attentiveness to Power and Its Influence on Relationships

A person's culture, gender, race, age, sexual orientation, physical condition, education, socioeconomic status, religion, and possible membership in other marginalized groups influence how power was granted to them based on their social location. As Freedman and Combs (1996) stated, some people have easier access to a wider range of sociocultural narratives than others and are entitled to more choices in their lives.

This explains the mixed experiences I encountered in the USA as they intersect with multiple social locations in my personal and professional journey (Hernandez & McDowell, 2010). Despite my marginalized identities as a Taiwanese female, I am privileged in terms of education, training, and vocation as an academia and supervisor in higher education. I work in an environment that often minimizes cultural traits that I value and are "innate" to me (e.g., being quiet and considerate, focusing on others' needs, and sacrificing without complaint); yet, I am in a power position that is reinforced by the academic structure. Because of cultural and gender social location, I am an "authority figure" that does not look, sound, or behave like my mainstream counterparts, and at times challenged by students. The postmodern approach's attentiveness to power and its influence on relationships provided an avenue to deepen my understanding of numerous relationships in which I feel comfortable and empowered as well as those that I feel "brushed off" and marginalized.

With this understanding, it is important to pay close attention to my relational use of power as an instructor and supervisor in the classroom. In order to be held accountable for proper use of this power and to monitor my personal "biases," I situate myself in a way that explicitly identifies my own experiences and intentions that influence clinical supervision and therapeutic work. For instance, I constantly reflect on the reasons why I choose a certain theory or suggest a specific intervention to the student. Although this self-work is not highlighted in postmodern supervision, it is important for me as a supervisor to regularly reflect on my biases in order to be clear about my positions, including my strengths and limitations, and to identify instances where my personal issues interfere with my professional work.

More often than not, this self-reflection process engages various social locations and identities, either in my private time or in peer consultation, within myself or with my professional colleagues. For example, conversations with my Asian colleagues and mentors "normalize" the contextual challenges a faculty of color faces; and consultations with my non-Asian colleagues and mentors provide a universal perspective that most instructors deal with in their classroom. I gained self-knowledge because of all of these dialogues and reflections and understand the complexities and profound influences of intersectionality and relational power within MFT supervision. It is only through understanding myself that I can appreciate the similarities and differences of others. Only through this self-work can I be aware of how my own life experiences and "bias" influence the ways I see and listen to my students. The postmodern lens opens the door to attend to the sociopolitical complications and power confusions. That aids in avoiding practices that subjugate others or capitalize on my power as an instructor and supervisor in the classroom. With this insight of my positional and relational power and the subsequent emotional comfort it brings, I am able to watch myself and to not overcompensate my "powerlessness" in certain aspects of my personal and professional life by abusing my power in supervisory relationships with students (Wilcoxon, Remley, & Gladding, 2014).

What Do I Do in Postmodern Supervision?

Meanings are constantly negotiated and cocreated among individuals, the others around them, and a larger cultural aggregation (Freedman & Combs, 1996). Supervision consists of an interpersonal and dynamic process of constructing and co-constructing realities of each student. In the following section, I will describe how I see myself applying concepts of postmodern supervision in MFT practicum classes and how my social location influences these interventions. I will also provide examples of how I use myself as a "cultural outsider" to promote students' awareness and learning about the influences of dominant discourses highlighted in the postmodern approach.

Decentering of the Dominant Professional Account of Knowledge

As a co-learner in the supervision process, I pay attention to the influences of power, social contexts, and the larger professional discourses within the supervisory relationship. Using a parallel process, I ask students similar questions and facilitate discussions to explore their own life trajectories relating to these diverse social indicators and their influence on personal and professional identities and clinical treatments. In doing so, a decentering of the dominant professional account of knowledge could happen, and trainees may become more familiar with their personal local knowledge that comes from the rich history of their life paths (Carlson & Erickson, 2001). When trainees see themselves as experts of their own stories, it is likely that they would adopt the belief that people are experts on their own lives and create spaces for clients to tell their own stories in the therapy room (Bobele, Biever, Solorzano, & Bluntzer, 2014).

A Not-Knowing Stance

I take a curious, not-knowing stance and inquire about the clinical meanings and connections my trainees make for case conceptualization. I have also offered my observations of the case and the influence of the trainees' social location on their clinical interpretation and therapeutic interaction in a personal and not intimidating way. For example, I have referred to my own social location and shared my perspective as a "cultural outsider," to explain how I see individualism and independence as one of the dominant cultural stories, and further describe ways in which I perceive these cultural stories as influencing the trainees' interventions or their clients' family dynamic. For instance, in a previous case consultation, a supervisee shared that her client is a 38-year-old Asian American male living with his older mother. Historically, American society has expected children to leave home when they reach adulthood, whereas traditional Taiwanese culture typically encourages adult children, especially sons, to co-reside with their older parents. In this case, interdependence is stressed more than independence in the parent-child relationship. I narrated very briefly about my own cultural and gendered story of my mom's desire for a son to take care of her when she is old, in order to help the trainees explore how the Western and Eastern cultural values may have informed their clinical judgments and the client's family life. Students reported it as insightful, while others seized the opportunity to "educate" me about the American culture. Mutually, we gained from these discussions as we coeducate each other. I make efforts to meet them through both differences and commonalities surrounding social locations.

Deconstructive Listening

Most of the time, I work with what my students present to me—their notes, stories, analyses, and selected therapy videos shared in a practicum class. Despite the standard case presentation components, students consciously or unconsciously choose certain materials and ways of narrating their therapeutic stories. It is important to explore this underlying process of "selection" and listen to both the said and unsaid. For example, every culture has its own dominant discourses and storylines. Discourses and storylines that are not the same as the mainstream are often discouraged in obvious or subtle ways. In other words, although there are multiple ways to narrate a client's life and therapeutic relationship, society provides only certain dominant narratives that are considered appropriate or relevant templates for describing or interpreting one's behaviors and experiences. These mainstream discourses define the client's and the student therapist's social roles and standards, such as the meaning of being a "good student" or being "successful." It is very likely that certain parts of clients' lives and trainees' experiences may be ignored, disapproved of, or oppressed by the dominant discourses while others remain unnoticed (Freedman & Combs, 1996; White, 1991).

Therefore, when listening to trainees' narratives in supervision, I apply deconstructive listening, that is, giving attention to the unnoticed or less-storied aspects, such as "struggles against injustice," strengths, or resources in clients' and trainees' lives (Freedman & Combs, 1996). I pay attention to the influence of restrictive cultural stories and the power distributions between the client family and the student therapist. I ask questions to help trainees unpack their accounts and see their current cases and interventions from a different perspective.

However, applying the stance of not-knowing, the intervention of deconstructive listening and the primarily conversational format of postmodern supervision present some unique challenges and learning opportunities. This collaborative and not-knowing role I assume presents a much less authoritative position compared with other theories. The preferred supervision style of inquiries, conversations, and discussions, instead of lectures and directive instructions, could be misunderstood as revealing me as "inexperienced" or suggesting that I "don't know" the answer. Acknowledging multiple possibilities and speaking softly could also be viewed as "not confident," "unsure," or "weak." As mentioned earlier, stereotypes of gender, age, and race might compound this first impression of incompetence.

This style of trainee-centered and decentering of the dominant professional account approach can be anxiety-provoking for beginning therapists, especially when they believe that I, as the supervisor, am responsible for providing a definite answer to the client's problem (Bobele et al., 2014). Some trainees might feel uneasy and uncomfortable adopting this style and even doubt the effectiveness of therapy and supervision. For instance, instead of viewing the stance of not-knowing as an intentional clinical intervention and supervision approach, the beginning therapist who did not receive the directive and straightforward instructions they expected from me may see this trainee-centered approach as a sign of me being an "inexperienced" and "incompetent" supervisor. Stereotypes associated with my marginalized identities (e.g., race and gender), again, might compound this impression of incompetence. Establishing credibility for me as a Taiwanese female postmodern MFT supervisor is a continuous effort when using the postmodern stance. As such, I found ways to make known my "expert" knowledge through sharing my training and education backgrounds, and referencing textbooks explicitly to "justify" my clinical suggestions with new students. Moreover, I responded to students' questions directly instead of redirecting to the class for varied viewpoints. This may not be my modus operandi but at times a necessary method in demonstrating the vast trainings and experiences I have.

Hierarchy and Collaboration

Despite the marginalized aspects of my identity, as a MFT supervisor, I am required to perform evaluations and make judgment of my supervisees' clinical progress and skills. The evaluative role associated with the supervisory position is inevitably attached to different kinds of power, such as legitimate power (e.g., the responsibility of evaluating, gatekeeping, grading, etc.) and relational power over supervisees (Wilcoxon et al., 2014). This power differential can be apparent, especially when working with beginning student therapists in their first practicum class. Some students seek and rely heavily on my guidance and advice. I am intentional about reducing the less helpful aspects of positional hierarchies and maximize the collaborative, cooperative, and mutual generation of ideas (Bobele et al., 2014).

For instance, when working with beginning therapists, I describe where my questions, comments, or observations come from and offer my intentions behind them, so, my students can better evaluate my "bias" and decide how to relate to it (Freedman & Combs, 2008). I situate my thoughts and ideas within the contexts in which I was raised, educated, and trained. Except for legal, ethical, or pressing clinical issues (e.g., crisis intervention), I present my recommendations as one way of conducting therapy but not the way of doing so. In doing this, I intend to create space for students' voices and to remain mindful of the power dynamic and "sociopolitical issues that can subtly direct the process" (Gehart & Tuttle, 2003, p. 216). As a result, my students take a more involved role in their professional development.

New and Alternative Stories

In supervisory practices, I use the insights and observations I gained through traveling and living in different cultures as well as my social location as a "cultural outsider," to challenge my students' assumptions and to raise their awareness of the dominant discourses. I use cultural conversations regarding our supervisory relationship to broaden their perspectives that are restricted by the mainstream narratives. In doing so, I facilitate the process of re-authoring new and alternative stories, which express ideas, thoughts, and emotions that have been suppressed by the negative societal narratives. Through this process, I attempt to bring forth and nurture "thick descriptions" and meaningful, multistranded stories that include different aspects of clients' lives and trainees' clinical work.

For instance, in a previous case consultation, a teenage client seemed very discouraged by being called a "nerd." My trainee's observation suggested that the client appeared introverted and lack social skills. He might have a negative self-image relating to being too "nerdy." During group supervision, we discussed the trainee's proposition for basic social skills training and also examined the meaning of "nerd" in client's social context and its implication on his interpersonal and family relationships. As a "cultural outsider," I shared that in some Asian cultures, in which children's academic performance is highly emphasized, there is actually a value attached to being a "nerd." Some parents even prefer their child to be "nerdy"— that is, to care less about social and physical attractiveness and focus merely on knowledge, school, and good grades. There might be varied interpretations of being "nerdy" in different industries (e.g., high-tech industry versus traditional manufacturing) and geographical locations (e.g., urban versus rural). The expansion of ideas was not to determine which cultural value is "right" or "better," but to open up a discussion about different possibilities and ways to look at the same "problem" (Freedman & Combs, 1996). Through constructing and reconstructing stories of as-yet-unstoried aspects, trainees may find new retelling of themselves as a therapist and as a person (Freedman & Combs, 2008). Many of my students were pleasantly surprised by this meaning-making process and strength-based approach.

Conclusion

My social location has influenced my journey to an academic position I am in today. My relationship with my mom was significant in constructing my narrative and my preferred way of performing my academic responsibilities, especially in clinical supervision. However, I know that my story as a Taiwanese female postmodern MFT supervisor working from a cross-cultural context will keep evolving and will be re-authored as I continue my journey in the discipline of MFT. I am excited about the years to come and am thankful for my friends and families as well as my compassionate, patient, and truthful mentors, colleagues, administrators, and many others who have supported me and created spaces for me when I am dealing with the challenges and power confusion as a female faculty of color. Without you, I could never have become me.

Acknowledgment To my strong-minded mom and loving husband who inspired me and pushed me through many life challenges; my mentors, supervisors, colleagues, and friends who have offered me your precious company, genuine support, and kind help; also everyone in the publishing team who have provided valuable feedback in my self-reflection and writing journey of this chapter. Special thanks to the editors for including me in this publication. I could never complete this chapter without each of you.

References

Anderson, H. (1997). *Conversation, language, and possibilities: A postmodern approach to therapy*. New York, NY: Basic Books.

Ashton, D., & Jordal, C. (2019). Revisioning gender, revisioning power: Equity, accountability, and refusing to silo. In M. McGoldrick & K. Hardy (Eds.), *Revisioning family therapy: Race, class, culture, and gender in clinical practice* (3rd ed.). New York, NY: Guilford Press.

Bobele, M., Biever, J. L., Solorzano, B. H., & Bluntzer, L. H. (2014). Postmodern approaches to supervision. In T. C. Todd & C. L. Storm (Eds.), *The complete systemic supervisor: Context, philosophy, and pragmatics* (pp. 255–273). Hoboken, NJ: John Wiley & Sons, Ltd..

Carlson, T., & Erickson, M. (2001). Honoring the privileging personal experience and knowledge: Ideas for a narrative therapy approach to the training and supervision of new therapists. *Contemporary Family Therapy, 23*(2), 199–219.

Crotty, M. (1998). *The foundations of social research*. Thousand Oaks, CA: SAGE Publications.

Fan, Y., Shepherd, L. J., Slavich, E., Waters, D., Stone, M., Abel, R., et al. (2019). Gender and cultural bias in student evaluations: Why representation matters. *PLoS One, 14*(2), e0209749. https://doi.org/10.1371/journal.pone.0209749.

Freedman, J., & Combs, C. (2008). Narrative couple therapy. In A. S. Gurman (Ed.), *Clinical handbook of couple therapy* (pp. 229–258). New York, NY: Guilford Press.

Freedman, J., & Combs, G. (1996). *Narrative therapy: The social construction of preferred realities*. New York, NY: Norton.

Gao, Y., Hu, D., Peng, E., Abbey, C., Ma, Y., Wu, C. I., et al. (2020). Depressive symptoms and the link with academic performance among rural Taiwanese children. *International Journal of Environmental Research and Public Health, 17*(8), 2778.

Gehart, D. R., & Tuttle, A. R. (2003). *Theory-based treatment planning for marriage and family therapy*. Pacific Grove, CA: Brooks/Cole.

Hernandez, P., & McDowell, T. (2010). Intersectionality, power, and relational safety in context: Key concepts in clinical supervision. *Training and Education in Professional Psychology, 4*, 29–35.

Hsieh, A. L., & Bean, R. A. (2014). Understanding familial/cultural factors in adolescent depression: A culturally competent treatment for working with Chinese American families. *American Journal of Family Therapy, 42*(5), 398–412.

Lee, E., & Mock, M. R. (2005a). Chinese families. In M. McGoldrick, J. Giordano, & N. Garcia-Preto (Eds.), *Ethnicity and family therapy* (pp. 269–289). New York, NY: Guilford Press.

Lee, E., & Mock, M. R. (2005b). Asian families: An overview. In M. McGoldrick, J. Giordano, & N. Garcia-Preto (Eds.), *Ethnicity and family therapy* (pp. 302–318). New York, NY: Guilford Press.

Quek, K. M., & Knudson-Martin, C. (2008). Reshaping marital power: How dual-career newlywed couples create equality in Singapore. *Journal of Social & Personal Relationships, 25*(3), 511–532.

Quek, K. M., Knudson-Martin, C., Orpen, S., & Victor, J. (2011). Gender equality during the transition to parenthood: A longitudinal study of dual-career couples in Singapore. *Journal of Social & Personal Relationships, 28*(7), 943–962.

Sue, D. W., & Sue, D. (2012). *Counseling the culturally diverse: Theory and practice* (6th ed.). Hoboken, NJ: John Wiley & Sons.

Walsh, F. (2019). Social class, rising inequality, and the American Dream. In M. McGoldrick & K. Hardy (Eds.), *Revisioning family therapy: Race, class, culture, and gender in clinical practice* (3rd ed.). New York, NY: Guilford Press.

White, M. (1991). Deconstruction and therapy. *Dulwich Center Newsletter, 3*, 21–40.

Wilcoxon, A. P., Remley, T. P., & Gladding, S. T. (2014). *Ethical, legal, and professional issues in the practice of marriage and family* (5th ed.). Boston, MA: Pearson.

Chapter 8
Dismantling Whiteness to Direct a Just Couples and Family Therapy Program: Experiences of a White Program Director

Christie Eppler

I asked the editors if I could title my chapter, Let Me White Woman That. To "White woman" something is to have the ascribed ability to take action, often at the expense of others due to a lack of awareness regarding implicit biases and privilege. Internet memes illustrate White "Karens" and "Beckys" attempting to solve problems with organized planning and a passion for enforcing their rules. At their worst, they ask to speak to a manager if food is not delivered fast enough, even during a pandemic (Greig, 2020). As a seasoned therapist, it is easy to telegraph that using a coy title was a reflection of not wanting to write or talk about justice, privilege, diversity, and inclusion, or an expression of my White fragility and guilt (DiAngelo, 2018; Swim & Miller, 1999). Yet, this proposed title aligns with what makes me successful as a program director of a Commission on the Accreditation of Marriage and Family Therapy Education (COAMFTE) accredited master's degree. When I think about my leadership style, many of my White woman traits come in handy. Spend my summer bossing around a 157-page self-study? Check. Double-checking national exam and curriculum alignment? Check. Nudging, cajoling, and nagging faculty so that rubrics are published in syllabi and collected at the end of each quarter? Check. Often, I ask myself if my White woman processes can live in peace with what is really important to me: being an ally, striving to decolonize the profession, and leading a socially just couples and family therapy program.

This chapter is not specifically about directing a marriage and family therapy (MFT) accredited program or what is necessary to decolonize the profession; rather, this chapter is my story of being a White, cis-female, heterosexual, able-bodied, middle-aged program director. There are excellent articles and texts that have explicated the importance of deconstructing Whiteness in systemic therapy (Baima & Sude, 2020), advocating for intersectionality (Dee Watts-Jones, 2010), contextual

C. Eppler (✉)
Couples and Family Therapy, Seattle University, Seattle, WA, USA
e-mail: epplerc@seattleu.edu

© Springer Nature Switzerland AG 2021   81
K. M.-T. Quek, A. L. Hsieh (eds.), *Intersectionality in Family Therapy Leadership*, AFTA SpringerBriefs in Family Therapy,
https://doi.org/10.1007/978-3-030-67977-4_8

and multicultural clinical approaches (Almeida, 2019; D'Arrigo-Patrick, Hoff, Knudson-Martin, & Tuttle, 2017; Falicov, 2014; Hernández, Siegel, & Almeida, 2009; Lebow, 2019; McDowell, 2005; McDowell, Knudson-Martin, & Bermudez, 2019; Parker, 2008), and augmenting social justice-related MFT research (Imber-Black, 2011; Seedall, Holtrop, & Parra-Cardona, 2014). This chapter, steeped in the literature, describes my experiences as an ally and program director who strives to be critically conscious (McDowell & Jeris, 2004). With hope, my words will honor and challenge the profession I have dedicated myself to for over 20 years.

The originators of systemic therapy rejected the medical model (Eppler, 2018) and were the mavericks of psychotherapy (Daneshpour, 2016). As a profession that long considered context but privileged White voices, there has been progress in synthesizing social-political constructs with assessment, conceptualization, and treatment (Almeida, 2019; Falicov, 2014). There is a robust account of training therapists to be mindful of social location (Hardy & Bobes, 2016; Hernandez-Wolfe & McDowell, 2012; McGoldrick et al., 1999; Winston & Piercy, 2010). While many program directors agree that diversity and inclusion are important, issues of justice are overshadowed by the priority given to dominant cultural narratives, including the focus on numeric outcomes, jockeying for economic resources, and other capitalist or categorical pursuits (e.g., reporting benchmarks, graduation rates, and licensure statistics).

While it is possible to have a systemic therapy training program that strives toward justice, we must ask if our structures promote or are barriers to training systemic therapists who embody justice. Is it possible to decolonize the profession while inducting students into an established field? The most pressing question of my career is: How can we enhance the dialogue and action regarding infusing social justice into systemic training programs while maintaining COAMFTE accreditation, high Association of Marriage and Family Therapy Regulatory Boards (AMFTRB) pass rates, and graduating new therapists who are prepared to work in the field? At times, I feel that the two realms—social justice and criteria set by the Department of Education and other regulatory boards—are too far apart for synthesis. But the mavericks of family therapy would eschew this linear thinking and find a way forward, would they not?

Let Me White Woman That

I am really White. My German and English ancestors were early colonizers of the United States. When I was an adolescent, a friend asked if I was wearing white pantyhose when I was not. I grew up in the 1980s in the suburban part of Kansas that borders on the rural. It was a place of vast fields and new shopping malls. I attended a conservative Christian church where, although few would admit to watching the television program "Dallas," we were informed by the styles and the ethos of the series' cliques, competition, and glamour. Not having the lavish life shown on television, I was taught that hard work led to fruitful outcomes. The code was clear: If you worked hard enough, you would be fine. "I'm fine" is still my automatic response to a myriad of questions—so much so that when my appendix burst, I told myself that I was fine until colleagues asked me to go to the hospital immediately.

This "I'm fine" attitude combined with the belief that hard work leads to positive outcomes was a barrier to my understanding of oppression and injustice, as it was easy to attribute success and failure to effort and determination or a lack thereof. Growing up, I never considered the unequal structures that support White people's success (Wise, 2011). In a high school pottery class, I remember the teacher talking about the growing homeless population. He opined that if the poor got jobs, they would not be homeless. No one asked about structural barriers to accessing resources. No one discussed what it would be like to work hard to find a job only to be turned down based on factors beyond one's control (e.g., skin color, ability to hire someone to vet a resume).

In order to unlearn the effects of racism and become aware of implicit biases, I had to learn about my Whiteness and privilege (Akamatsu, 2008; Combs, 2019; Helms, 2017). It was important to admit that being fine by working hard was due in large part to the invisible structures that supported my success. It was not until the end of my graduate studies that I first heard about White privilege (McIntosh, 1988). A White doctoral student in an adjacent program spoke often about her unearned privilege. In a seminar, she gave a presentation during which she brought in symbols from throughout her life that represented invisible benefits she received on account of being White. She placed a resume at the top of a stack while highlighting that her European name, her suburban address, and her previous degrees elevated her resume to the top. While she was confident in her abilities, she was also aware that a system of power elevated her resume above those who did not share this unearned privilege.

When I examined the fruits of my hard work, I transformed from a linear perspective—hard work leads to payoffs—to acknowledging that I too have benefited from invisible structures and systemic privilege. I acknowledged that my Whiteness afforded me opportunities for positive outcomes even when I did not work hard. There have been grades that were higher than deserved, likely because I am nice, I try, and most importantly, I am White, heterosexual, cis-female, temporarily able-bodied, middle class, and born in the United States. My experiences are echoed in Baima and Sude's (2020) study's findings about what mental health professionals need to know about Whiteness. Like the participants, I had to work to become aware, transformed, and move through uncomfortable feelings about race and ethnicity.

My first full-time academic job was in northern New Jersey, which was a more racially and ethnically diverse environment than I had experienced previously. I was a young scholar, not yet 30. I remember feeling like a fledgling when a student twice my age told me to get off my high horse because she did not agree with my recommendation. Although my age positioned me to feel less powerful, I had ascribed power as a White person and an assistant professor. I started to understand that power was multilayered and dynamic, changing in situations and throughout my development.

I taught students from across social locations and I made mistakes. For example, I was a reader for a Black student's dissertation, and after a heated conversation, which I had interpreted as having rude elements, the student talked with me about cultural communication styles (Sue, 2015). I was able to shift my perspective from an embedded belief that productive conversations are quiet and polite to realizing that there are multiple forms of respectful, collaborative, and productive expression. I am now able to name that it was not my Black student's responsibility to teach me (Watson, 2016), and I am grateful that she did.

Early in my career, I transitioned from New Jersey to the Pacific Northwest to teach in a counselor educator program, which stands on settled land belonging to First Nation communities, including the Duwamish tribe. I returned to classrooms that were mostly White and female. I felt the loss of vibrant and diverse conversations with multiple perspectives. I received criticism from faculty and students who did not appreciate my stance that understanding diversity starts with self-reflection (Akamatsu, 2008; Baima & Sude, 2020; Combs, 2019; Helms, 2017). Meanwhile, I connected with many students from underrepresented backgrounds who found it refreshing that I considered issues of justice.

Six years later, I moved to a university across town to return to teaching systemic therapy. I worked alongside a Black male director who had a rich professional history but less knowledge of accreditation standards. I quickly found myself feeling my "let me White woman that" tendencies as we worked to achieve accreditation. I became intimately familiar with revised standards, and I felt like the new kid eschewing the established procedures to modernize and Whitewash the program. I feared that my changes would be interpreted as microaggressions (Sue, 2015). Just before our program achieved accreditation, the former director retired, and I was appointed to his position. Now, with even more ascribed power, I had to increase how I intentionally connect with students, staff, and faculty.

Womanist Leadership

One surprise that came with being director is that my students viewed me as a director trope instead of who I am. They saw in me a hologram of their previous experiences of people in power, which were likely shaped by patriarchal experiences. In their minds, I was aloof, intimidating, and unapproachable. I wanted to say, "Last week—before I became the director—you saw me as caring and relatable." I heard that students did not want to meet with me because I was busy; my interpretation of their rationale was that they were scared of me. I had full daily agendas, but I never asked a student to wait more than a few days for a requested appointment. When meeting with students from minoritized backgrounds, they were understandably surprised when I took their concerns seriously. In my 5 years of being a director, I have tried to listen intently and make as many decisions as possible collaboratively, even if it took more time and energy than making choices superficially or unilaterally. For example, a White male student wanted to switch supervision groups. Our groups are closed, but another student was willing to change. Before allowing the transfer, I asked both groups, the entire cohort, to meet and discuss the ramifications. When students wondered aloud why this was not an easy choice, I asked them to contemplate the power structures and justice issues underneath the seemingly simple decision.

My core values of humility, curiosity, perseverance, and taking a nonanxious and not-knowing stance are critical to my womanist leadership. When situations are fraught, I often ask myself what I could have done differently. If my White woman heritage is to be a fixer without having the power of male privilege, then I am left to center myself as the target for what needs to be changed. Self-reflection is a humble practice, and there are times when I realize that I am not the epicenter of the problem. My marriage and family therapy training encourages me to be curious and ask questions, especially when anxiety is high. When students, staff, and faculty share concerns with me—which can be about solvable problems, situations that I do not have the power to change, or issues that they themselves need to work through to promote their professional development—I channel Bowen's ideas about taking a nonanxious stance (Bowen, 1978) and root myself in visions of empowerment of self and others. I navigate being relational while at times having to toe the party line. All the while, I remain aware of the larger systems that can impede change and justice.

Barriers to Just Leadership

The prevalent structure that affects my directorship is COAMFTE. There are many standards and key elements in COAMFTE's version 12 that address diversity and antidiscrimination. These requirements are important, yet they are only a small part of what is needed to decolonize the profession. Accreditation is a classification system, a Western concept of determining fit and value. While it may be impossible for marriage and family therapy educators to eschew accreditation, work is needed to enhance how social justice is woven into training programs. The world of achievement, correct punctuation, and checking boxes is the dominant and demanding voice in my professional life, and I find that my passion for social justice often takes a back seat as I maintain my program's accreditation.

When I entered the realm of accreditation, I thought naively that the process would dovetail with MFT's strength-based, contextually focused, collaborative ethos. I attended expensive accreditation seminars, during which I read my student learning outcomes aloud to a working group with a representative who indicated that my program's objectives were acceptable. However, the official critique rebuffed our outcomes and indicated that my program did not utilize the authorized, yet unpublished template. Our self-study was determined to be insufficient. After hiring a consultant and resubmitting our application without making substantive changes to the program, we achieved accreditation.

This process raised questions about justice since it required significant economic resources and submission to the dominant narrative. I wondered if a program director must be an insider or know insiders in order to speak the official language and be accredited. I worried that this process was one example of how the dominant culture protects the dominant culture. I heard from supportive others who have been through the process successfully, "Here is what they want, because they won't tell you what they really want." Other program directors commiserated with me when our program's review feedback exceeded the expectations listed. We opined about the amount of busy work it took to remain accredited. And we joked that programs are held to a higher standard than COAMFTE itself, as the commission does not publish outcome data to verify that graduates from accredited programs are better therapists than graduates from healthy but nonaccredited programs.

Through these conversations, I gained deeper empathy for people on the margins and an enhanced understanding of systemic privilege (e.g., having the economic resources, access to other directors in position of power). Although I am wary of the potential for accreditation to inhibit social justice progress, I am not calling for COAMFTE to be dismantled, as there is a place for quality assurance. However, this control should not supersede a vision of inclusive, diverse education that prioritizes marginalized voices.

At the time my program sought initial accreditation, I was a tenured associate professor. Thus, I had fewer responsibilities than a junior academic (e.g., less pressure to publish and fewer new course preparations). As a White academic, I did not have additional duties required of faculty from minoritized backgrounds, such as mentoring students of color and being appointed the unofficial diversity representative on university committees (DeWelde & Stepnick, 2015). While the profession must have faculty from diverse backgrounds in positions of power, we first have to consider how COAMFTE requirements that consume time, energy, and other resources affect minoritized faculty members' professional development, given the unequal and unwritten expectations placed on them (Chun & Evans, 2014; DeWelde & Stepnick, 2015). I desire to hire a full-time faculty member from a minoritized background to codirect the program (i.e., divide the workload so that a faculty person of color is not overburdened with administration, regular faculty expectations, and the emotional energy of being a faculty of color). Regrettably, my advocacy for a tenure-track line has yet to be successful. Meanwhile, I appreciate the grassroots efforts that program directors have made toward mentoring junior faculty, and my work is to help memorialize these mechanisms of support within official structures. And, it is imperative for me to continue to connect with existing resources that support inclusion of diverse therapists and future leaders (e.g., AAMFT's Minority Fellowship Program, Counselors of Color Regional Network).

Building Just Connections

Collaborating, mentoring, and co-teaching build connections among faculty from diverse social locations. Creating a strong rapport is important to facilitating justice-oriented faculty meetings, where there are often differences. I am grateful for core and adjunct faculty who embrace dedicating faculty meetings to discussing justice, even if we are at different points in our cultural attunement journeys and we do not always agree. For example, in one meeting, we discussed preferred terms and definitions. For instance, do we refer to "students of color," "minoritized students," or "underrepresented students"? We did not reach a consensus. Likewise, there was a significant discussion when some faculty members advocated for prioritizing the needs of Black and Brown people, which Asian American faculty experienced as marginalization of themselves and their communities.

Moreover, we do not agree on being called by our first names versus formal titles. Preston (2016) used queer theory to explore how students should address their professors. Preston began their career by being on a first name basis with students as an act to ameliorate hierarchy. However, they transitioned to being called by their professional title to increase the transparency of classroom power dynamics. For now, with the encouragement of my faculty from Latinx and Black backgrounds, I have chosen to go by Dr. Eppler. However, I know that going by my title has an effect on how students relate to me as an "unapproachable" director.

As program director, I seek to ensure that all faculty have a voice and are heard by one another. As a White person, I monitor how much space I take up in conversations to break the cultural pattern of privileging White voices. At times, my silence may come across as an act of White guilt (DiAngelo, 2018). It has been difficult for me to navigate the balance of leading and listening. My commitment is to be overt about naming that I do not want to dominate the conversation. I am mindful that to be able to say, "I do not want to dominate the conversation" reminds me of my privilege. Hence, I have increased active listening and sitting with the discomfort of not having easy answers and immediate solutions.

In my own journey of being mentored, I have been fortunate to work with and learn from faculty from minoritized backgrounds. One of the best professional experiences of my career was co-teaching with a Latinx academic. I witnessed how she brought conversations about diversity to life by talking about her embodied experiences, which contrasts with the more cognitive understanding I have about oppression, racism, and injustice. Chun and Evans (2014) advocated that universities need to allot additional resources to bolster knowledge and skills related to diversity and inclusion. When my colleague and I co-taught, we each received half credit toward our teaching loads, although it was not half the work (i.e., both instructors were present for all class sessions, we both graded all assignments). Similarly, when hiring mentors of color to support White faculty to develop cultural humility, I have been successful in securing small stipends. However, additional funds are needed to build collaborative and transformative experiences. It is becoming increasingly challenging to secure funds for this critical work.

I value reciprocal relationships, and my team has taught me much about being a director and working with people across social locations. Faculty have given me excellent advice when working with students from underrepresented backgrounds. Specifically, faculty from minoritized backgrounds suggested that I need to give students of color clear and concrete directions. While I value being transparent, my systems training guides me toward the ethereal, and my natural tendency is to think of empowerment in terms of leaving space for others' creativity. I now understand how this can be difficult for those who are coming into a system that is foreign to them. I continue to struggle to balance being appropriately direct with not wanting to indoctrinate students into the status quo. I am learning to be clear while leaving room for new voices who will transform the profession. To do so, I paradoxically step back and provide mentoring from a culturally humble position.

Believing in the power of mentoring, I prioritize supporting my faculty. However, given my privilege, I hold potential to further the dominant narrative. To mediate this risk, I ask that all faculty uphold a dedication to diversity by using gender-inclusive language, assigning readings by underrepresented and minoritized authors, and taking a stance of curiosity and compassion when differences arise. To enhance justice in my program, I demonstrate the importance of taking a growth mindset, showing by example that it is critical to learn and grow from mistakes, especially when there are missteps related to internalized racism. I consider equality, equity, and how actions affect the entire system. It is important for me to listen to faculty and trust their expertise. I give my faculty a wide berth so that they may have both autonomy and support. When students complain, I talk directly with faculty and listen to their perspectives.

Even when I employ the mechanisms listed above, challenging situations arise. For example, an instructor from a marginalized background taught a pre-practicum class utilizing a strength-based and critically conscious lens. One of their goals was to assist students from minoritized backgrounds in liberating themselves from oppressive structures by encouraging them to trust their inner voices and push back against being acculturated into a White profession. While this was imperative for students of color to hear, students from the dominant culture internalized these messages of empowerment through their privileged lenses. Subsequent faculty noted that White students were not utilizing instructor feedback. When asked about this, White students cited the pre-practicum instructor's recommendations to trust their intuition and be wary of oppressive voices. White students could not distinguish structural oppression from professional judgments made by a diverse faculty team. Before offering the next course, I met with the instructor. I had several constructs swirling in my thoughts: How could I empower the instructor to teach from their knowledge and experience (e.g., critical consciousness) while differentiating between how minoritized and dominant culture students receive the information? Were there parts of my White privilege that wanted to suppress the critical conscious focus of their class? What was best for all students (equality), and especially students of color who needed to hear empowering messages (equity)? What were structural barriers that influenced the situation (e.g., students scoring minoritized faculty lower on teaching evaluations could influence the decision to evaluate only strengths)?

To facilitate growth-oriented conversations, my job is to ask questions, listen to multiple perspectives, and dismantle the effects of my Whiteness by creating space for diverse voices. However, I believe that too much openness is detrimental to a healthy system. Thus, I determined that boundaries were needed for our learning community. My essential teaching practices are that faculty must bring their whole socially located selves into the classroom while supporting the development of students through respect and trauma-informed care. I encourage instructors to teach to transgress (Hooks, 1994) from a place of love (Hooks, 2018). Students, especially students who have experienced marginalization, have faced significant hurdles on the path to graduate school. They may be scarred or wounded. In contrast, students from the dominant culture may not have learned about power and privilege yet. A clinical training program must honor all students' pasts and futures.

In my program, instructors must utilize a growth mindset, wherein students are held responsible for their development. I recognized that many incoming students had yet to study liberation, inclusion, and social location. Thus, I moved our multi-cultural course to the first quarter of the program. This sets the program's positionality and sets a trajectory for students to be held accountable for recognizing their privilege. A lack of growth in cultural humility is grounds for remediation. I lament that faculty of color must endure students' inevitable pitfalls on the journey to becoming aware of themselves as cultural beings and attuned therapists (e.g., experiencing microaggressions before students develop multicultural awareness and skills).

I often tell my students that couples and family therapists are a people of tough and transformative conversations. We may not exit conversations in agreement, but each person needs to be seen and understood fully as a whole being. Conversations can be difficult, especially when students bring their backgrounds, passions, and beliefs into discussions. I remind myself and my faculty that students are in the program because they want to learn, grow, and be challenged.

Conclusion

It is important for me to talk with students and faculty about our current place in the history of MFT. I want them to celebrate how we have been the mavericks of mental health. And I want them to grieve our history of conceptualizing clients through a White gaze, which has been a disservice and harmful to clients from diverse backgrounds. I affirm that I—that we—are on a never-ending journey of cultural learning. I acknowledge my privilege and I articulate a commitment to eradicating White fragility by talking about social locations in the program, in classes, and in the larger couples and family therapy community. My conversation about justice and dismantling White privilege will be a continued dialogue.

I am grateful for my training and career as a couples and family therapist while acknowledging that I have been a White voice in a predominately White profession (Baima & Sude, 2020). I see my life's work as exploring, witnessing, and cultivating resilience and justice. I love when my faculty, staff, and students have significant "Aha!" moments related to multicultural growth. I have seen underrepresented students find their voices and thrive. And there have been challenging situations in which we could not comprehend or overcome the visible and invisible effects of racism and bias.

Becoming a systemic therapist and being a program director have heightened my sense of empathy for the marginalized, affirmed my commitment to see strengths in all, and cultivated my passion for justice. Being a couples and family therapist has made me a better ally, and my passion for social justice is enlivened because I see the world through a systemic lens. I would be a different leader if I were not also a licensed marriage and family therapist. Although the two jobs are distinct, I am able to draw on my training as I confront the challenges and joys of directing a just clinical training program.

Acknowledgments I thank the late Dr. Chantel Lumpkin and the late Dr. Monica Moutin Sanders, Black women who planted seeds of justice during my doctoral program at Michigan State University before I became intentional about dismantling my Whiteness. I would also like to thank Dr. Jodie Knott, who introduced me to the concept of White privilege. I am grateful for my core faculty, Drs. Jeanette Rodriguez, Jeney Park-Hearn, and Rebecca Cobb (who subverts the cultural narrative by being ally Becky).

References

Akamatsu, N. (2008). Teaching white students about racism and its implications in practice. In M. McGoldrick & K. V. Hardy (Eds.), *Re-visioning family therapy* (2nd ed., pp. 413–424). New York, NY: Guilford Press.

Almeida, R. V. (2019). *Liberation based healing practices*. NJ: Institute for Family Services.

Baima, T., & Sude, M. E. (2020). What White mental health professionals need to understand about Whiteness: A Delphi study. *Journal of Marital & Family Therapy, 46*(1), 62–80. https://doi-org.proxy.seattleu.edu/10.1111/jmft.12385.

Bowen, M. (1978). *Family therapy in clinical practice*. New York, NY: Jason Aronson.

Chun, E. B., & Evans, A. (2014). *The department chair as transformative leader: Building inclusive learning environments in higher education*. Sterling, VA: Stylus.

Combs, G. (2019). White privilege: What's a family therapist to do? *Journal of Marital and Family Therapy, 45*(1), 61–75. https://doi.org/10.1111/jmft.12330.

D'Arrigo-Patrick, J., Hoff, C., Knudson-Martin, C., & Tuttle, A. (2017). Navigating critical theory and postmodernism: Social justice and therapist power in family therapy. *Family Process, 56*, 574–588. https://doi.org/10.1111/famp.12236.

Daneshpour, M. (2016). Keynote address. In *American Association of marriage and family therapy national conference*, Atlanta, GA.

Dee Watts-Jones, T. (2010). Location of self: Opening the door to dialogue on intersectionality in the therapy process. *Family Process, 49*, 405–420. https://doi.org/10.1111/j.1545-5300.2010.01330.x.

DeWelde, K., & Stepnick, A. (2015). *Disrupting the culture of silence: Confronting gender inequality and making change in higher education.* Sterling, VA: Stylus.

DiAngelo, R. (2018). *White fragility.* Boston, MA: Beacon Press.

Eppler, C. (2018). Ecosystem in family systems theory. In J. L. Lebow, A. L. Chambers, & D. Breunlin (Eds.), *Encyclopedia of couple and family therapy.* Cham, Switzerland: Springer International Publishing.

Falicov, C. J. (2014). *Latino families in therapy* (2nd ed.). New York, NY: Guilford Press.

Greig, J. (2020, May 13). A Pennsylvania Karen attacked a Red Lobster employee over having to wait too long for her food. *Blavity:News.* Retrieved from: https://blavity.com/a-pennsylvania-karen-attacked-a-red-lobster-employee-over-having-to-wait-too-long-for-her-food?category1=news.

Hardy, K. V., & Bobes, T. (2016). *Culturally sensitive supervision and training: Diverse perspectives and practical applications.* New York, NY: Routledge.

Helms, J. E. (2017). The challenge of making whiteness visible: Reactions to four whiteness articles. *The Counseling Psychologist, 45*(5), 717–726. https://doi.org/10.1177/0011000017718943.

Hernández, P., Siegel, A., & Almeida, R. (2009). How does the cultural context model facilitate therapeutic change? *Journal of Marital and Family Therapy, 35,* 97–110.

Hernandez-Wolfe, P., & McDowell, T. (2012). Speaking of privilege: Family therapy educators' journeys towards awareness and compassionate action. *Family Process, 51*(2), 163–178. https://doi.org/10.1111/j.1545-5300.2012.01394.x.

Hooks, B. (1994). *Teaching to transgress: Education as the practice of freedom.* New York, NY: Routledge.

Hooks, B. (2018). *All about love: New visions.* New York, NY: Harper Prennial.

Imber-Black, E. (2011). Toward a contemporary social justice agenda in family therapy research and practice. *Family Process, 50,* 129–131. https://doi.org/10.1111/j.1545-5300.2011.01350.x.

Lebow, J. (2019). Editorial: Social justice in family therapy. *Family Process, 58*(1), 3–8. https://doi.org/10.1111/famp.12430.

McDowell, T. (2005). Practicing with a critical multicultural lens. *Journal of Systemic Therapies, 24,* 1–4.

McDowell, T., & Jeris, L. (2004). Talking about race using Critical Race Theory: Recent trends in the Journal of Marital and Family Therapy. *Journal of Marital and Family Therapy, 30,* 81–94.

McDowell, T., Knudson-Martin, C., & Bermudez, J. (2019). Third-order thinking in family therapy: Addressing social justice across family therapy practice. *Family Process, 58*(1), 9–22. https://doi.org/10.1111/famp.12383.

McGoldrick, M., Almeida, R., Preto, N., Bibb, A., Sutton, C., Hudak, J., et al. (1999). Efforts to incorporate social justice perspectives into a family training program. *Journal of Marital and Family Therapy, 25*(2), 191–209. https://doi.org/10.1111/j.1752-0606.1999.tb01122.x.

McIntosh, P. (1988). White privilege and male privilege: A personal account of coming to see correspondences through work in women's studies. *Working paper No. 189.* Wellesley, MA: Wellesley Center for Research on Women.

Parker, L. (2008). The cultural context model: A case study of social justice-based clinical practice. *Social Justice in Context, 3,* 25–40.

Preston, C. J. (2016, November 02). Do you make them call you 'professor'? *Chronical of Higher Education.* https://www.chronicle.com/article/Do-You-Make-Them-Call-You/238282.

Seedall, R. B., Holtrop, K., & Parra-Cardona, J. R. (2014). Diversity, social justice, and intersectionality trends in C/MFT: A content analysis of three family therapy journals, 2004–2011. *Journal of Marital and Family Therapy, 40*(2), 139–151. https://doi.org/10.1111/jmft.12015.

Sue, D. W. (2015). *Race talk and the conspiracy of silence: Understanding and facilitating difficult dialogues on race.* Hoboken, NJ: Wiley & Sons Inc..

Swim, J. K., & Miller, D. L. (1999). White guilt: Its antecedents and consequences for attitudes toward affirmative action. *Personality and Social Psychology Bulletin, 25*(4), 500–514. https://doi.org/10.1177/0146167299025004008.

Watson, M. (2016). Supervision in Black and White: Navigating cross-racial interactions in the supervisory process. In K. V. Hardy & T. Bobes (Eds.), *Culturally sensitive supervision and training: Diverse perspectives and practical applications* (pp. 43–49). New York, NY: Routledge.

Winston, E. J., & Piercy, F. P. (2010). Gender and diversity topics taught in commission on accreditation for marriage and family therapy education programs. *Journal of Marital and Family Therapy, 36*(4), 446–471. https://doi.org/10.1111/j.1752-0606.2010.00220.x.

Wise, T. (2011). *White like me*. Berkeley, CA: Soft Skull Press.

Chapter 9
What We Have Learned: Different Locations, Shared Experiences

Alexander Lin Hsieh and Karen Mui-Teng Quek

In this collection of personal essays, the MFT academic leaders examine the intersectionality of their social location, where differing social positions reinforce and interact with opportunity, power, marginalization, and discrimination. Multiple reciprocal influences are reflected in our lived experiences as MFT professors. The authors who have been in MFT academia, defined as education, supervision, and administration, between 5 and 20 years are attentive to issues of power and disadvantages in various academic and clinical settings. We see how these MFT leaders weave together their stories of achievement and discrimination. Each leader reflects on their commitment to social change and openness to continue in this type of work to support other faculty, professionals, and students in similar situations. Though each author's story is unique and profoundly inspiring, many commonalities connect the authors together and convey a larger story. The larger story as suggested in the title of this book "*Intersectionality in Family Therapy Leadership—Professional Power, Personal Identities*" is about MFT educators' collective encountering of inequality and discrimination as a result of our social locations and our greater access to power and resources that we used in initiating social change within our sphere of influence. We are not alone in these encounters, but with collective action through sharing experiences with colleagues, we gain success in our professional work.

In this concluding chapter, we want to highlight what we have learned. In particular, we will underscore the themes of visibility/invisibility, intersections of both oppressed and privileged stories, the continuous internal dialogue and critical

A. L. Hsieh (✉)
Couple and Family Therapy Program, Alliant International University, Sacramento, CA, USA
e-mail: ahsieh@alliant.edu

K. M.-T. Quek
Marriage and Family Therapy Program, Biola University (Talbot School of Theology),
La Mirada, CA, USA

© Springer Nature Switzerland AG 2021
K. M.-T. Quek, A. L. Hsieh (eds.), *Intersectionality in Family Therapy Leadership*, AFTA SpringerBriefs in Family Therapy,
https://doi.org/10.1007/978-3-030-67977-4_9

reflection, and using privilege to support the marginalized. Although each author has vastly different social location characteristics, all found ways to utilize their social locations to make a deep impact within their social and academic environment. These personal essays brought to light the dynamics between the MFT leaders' position of power, multiple social locations, and the discourse of structural power and inequality that disadvantages certain groups, together creating a significant phenomenon shaping their work narratives and professional identities. Before turning to the commonalities, we summarize how each author contends with those issues.

As she recounts her experiences, Karen Quek views the multiplicity of social location as intricately linked to her leadership development process. She draws our attention to the challenges of discrimination and opportunities to respond differently, which have informed the shaping of a female leader of color. Her marginalized voice was either silenced or talked over. She was bypassed in many decision-making within the system. Now, she finds ways to deal with that by giving voice to those who appear voiceless. She mentors younger colleagues and students from differing backgrounds by providing an environment of stability and psychological safety so that their voices can be heard. Being in a position of power, she leads her program, where each story and each voice matters.

Alexander Hsieh's narrative combines his Taiwanese American male identity with the MFT profession that has challenged his cultural norms. This interaction has created an internal dialogue around the juxtaposition of his own racial and cultural identity, along with his academic position of power and marginalized communities. As Alexander reflects on the social power as an MFT program director and clinical director, he has to decide how that privileged opportunity is utilized to benefit students and communities who are marginalized. He reflects on the contrast between his own cultural values and how that might bias his interaction with his local community. So, the interaction between his cultural and gender values, his academic roles, and place of residency allows him to change the landscape of mental health, bit by bit, using that privilege to affect his community both on a micro and macro-level and to support and hold space for marginalized communities.

Narumi Tanaguichi's narrative examines how the layers of intersectionality are often confusing, and how having power influences her engagement with others. Over the course of her narrative, she reveals that intersectionality associated with her identity as an Asian, queer, and immigrant woman often makes her invisible, but her newly acquired power as a MFT program director offers visibility within the institution. Because power and visibility come with responsibility, she intends to take up space as often as she can—even if that is uncomfortable to her—and open up space for others who are invisible.

The Spanish phrase "*Sí, se puede*" that translates as "Yes, it can be done" is a collective mantra to motivate and inspire the underrepresented, educate students about social justice issues, and help students learn how to respect and even positively esteem those who are different from them. This is key to Sergio Pereyra's narrative. He draws on discourses about Latino masculinity, Mormonism, and academic culture to articulate how he overcomes discrimination, reveals his Mormon religion, and integrates himself into the professional guild. While he acknowledges that change is a constant in the education system, he endorses taking a not-knowing stance, striving to educate himself about others and remaining open to new knowledge. Sergio reflects on how the striving starts first with himself, but also how it contributes to marginalized communities. He concludes with "*Sí, se puede*" (we can) make changes when we have the heart and willingness to do so.

Gita Seshadri's chapter takes the reader on an internal processing journey from anxiety to confidence in her academic position. She shares how her assumed privilege and role confusion shape her journey of self-discovery and deepen her understanding of humility. The implicit messages from her South Asian background conflict with the not-so-subtle messages from her American experiences. In doing so, she recognizes on a deeper level the importance of exploring social intersectionality in her personal and professional life. She concluded that not undertaking this work would make the invisible even more hidden. Undertaking this work, as it relates to her journey, puts her on a course for humility, thoughtfulness for others, and leaving space for others' reflective responses. She concluded that she has grown more confident while limiting the impact anxiety has on the nature and quality of her professional path.

Chen Hao-Min's narrative delves deeply into power differences associated with culture and gender hierarchy embedded in the social cultural discourse and the profound impact on her professional trajectory and relationships in the workplace. In her narrative, she highlights the limit of social power due to gender inequality and structural racism. Her story of the love-hate relationship with her mother is embedded in a patriarchal societal structure. In a similar manner, she sees a parallel to the current academic structure, where her social location related to gender, culture, and immigrant background continues to be subjected to discrimination. As an educator who now holds a position of power, she takes a postmodern stance in her work to level power differences and promote the power of multiple perspectives.

As an ally for social justice, Christie Eppler, a White, cis-female, heterosexual, middle-aged program director, narrates intentionality in her work and employs growth-oriented conversations in order to gain deeper empathy for people on the margins and an enhanced understanding of systemic privilege. She acknowledges her privilege and articulates a commitment to eradicating White fragility by talking about social locations in the program, in classes, and in the larger couples and family therapy community. This conversation about justice and dismantling White privilege will be a continued dialogue.

Despite our diversity, our narratives indicate how ethnic, race, and gender inequalities affect what happens to us as educators, clinicians, and supervisors. We are aware of the possibilities of sexist and or racist treatments and structural racism and seek to promote an environment that celebrates differences and promotes a commitment to social justice. That commitment includes finding ways to deal with ongoing inequality and disadvantages so that we can move forward in our journeys. With access to professional power as educational leaders, we conscientiously seek to make a difference in promoting our junior colleagues and students who are starting out in the field.

Visibility and Invisibility

Visibility generates attention. That may be a fact of life and consistent across all forms of science. We often comment on the visible changes of the seasons with appreciation for the changing colors of leaves and the first snow, but rarely highlight the unseen like gravity or the transmission of sound. Socially, our interests peak when couples argue in public or when they exhibit excessive public displays of affection. Meanwhile, secure attachment, masking of insecurities, and emotional affairs are less visible and often need much more effort to bring to attention. The visible are often synonymous with speaking up, speaking loudly, taking charge, having grander stature, and sometimes being more forceful and confrontational. The invisible, on the other hand, tends to work in the background, display more humility and slow to boast, and are more likely to be marginalized. In social constructionist thought, visibility is a privilege while marginalization leads to invisibility (Christensen, 2019). Our various intersectionality of sexual, gender, ethnic, and immigrant identities open us up to be increasingly invisible. While the literature argues that power and privilege bring about visibility, most leaders in these chapters speak on how each balances this visibility with their marginalized invisibilities. In addition, visibility creates a layer of burden for MFT leaders to use the privileged visibility to bring about positive change for the disadvantaged and the marginalized.

The theme of visibility versus invisibility is commonplace across the various chapters. Many of the authors acknowledged and shared instances of invisibility, but also instances where their social location allowed for heightened visibility. Narumi's positionality as a program director grants visibility, while her identity intersection as an Asian, queer, immigrant woman subjects her to being invisible. Similarly, Karen's experience of invisibility to an administrator leads her to create more visibility to faculty and educators of color so that diversity and multiculturalism is highlighted rather than an afterthought. Hao-Min's power-differential experience based on the subjection of the dominant discourse to her minority narrative impacts how she skillfully navigates her professional relationships to create more visibility within her program. Meanwhile, Hao-Min also has to overcome her own cultural invisibility built on cultural hierarchy to create her own personal agency and garner more visibility. Finally, Gita's professor status provides visibility, which she uses in conjunction with her collectivistic qualities like humility, work ethic, and consideration of others to clear a more visible professional path.

Often, visibility and invisibility are determined by social location and can change when someone's social location changes. Visibility plays a key role in how we carry out our responsibilities in academia, especially from the perspective of administration. While operating as an educator and supervisor might demonstrate a clear leadership figure, administrative roles often operate behind the scenes and away from the public eye. Because administrative roles may not always be at the forefront, they may be more invisible. While we are all visible in the professional world by various physical traits, other qualities, such as SES, sexual orientation, faith traditions, and nationality, are less so. These invisibilities may become more prominent with social interaction through experiences of racial and sexual discrimination, external pressures of interpersonal context to conform through traditional social norms, and microaggressions within racial communities. Faculty of color discussed the intertwining of gender, racial, and national identities and how these categories interacted to inform how we were perceived by the dominant culture. While visibility allows us to be heard and to be accountable to our positional power in the academe, invisibility may present a challenge to a freer expression of ourselves due to the need to protect self, to maintain a professional status quo, and to avoid any conflictual situations.

Intersections of Oppressed and Privileged Stories

There is power when stories are told. When narratives are shared from the first-person perspective, it gives the reader a firsthand account of events, personal history, the internal dialogue, and instantaneous reactions. These stories, at times, may be difficult to write just as much as it can be to read. The authors interwove intimate stories of oppression and stories where they gain greater access to opportunities and upward mobility. Stories of privileges and oppressions were sometimes confusing and conflicting. In Narumi's account, telling her story of intersecting identities and her path to the position of a program director, while confusing, creates visibility not only for her, but queer women in similar positions. Sergio's internal dialogue concerning his struggle and fit in the academe as a junior professor with diverse social identities brings about support to marginalized populations. Alexander's articulation of his privilege associated with the professional position as program director and his Asian identity, which is oppressed within the larger societal context, shape his passion for the underserved and increases his social responsibility for the local community. Hao-Min's navigation of the gendered constraints that shape her relationship with her mother has also led to more personal agency and built an incredible sense of resiliency, leading her to be a stronger leader for her students. As Gita tells her story, she gains confidence to draw on what can be seen as contradictory identities while decreasing levels of anxiety to clear a more distinct path in her professional journey and how she can impact her students.

Telling stories of oppression opens individuals up to many of our most vulnerable experiences. Many times, individuals who are in positions of power have difficulties being vulnerable because institutional cultural beliefs suggest that vulnerability gives away power and opens ourselves up to weakness. In reality, research has shown that vulnerability helps us build character and relationships and empowers us to gain control of our shame (Brown, 2012). Although there were many moments of silent pain, hurt, and suffering throughout each of our stories, our struggle and eventual rise from those anguished oppressions ultimately gives the authors strength and courage to meet the next challenge. Each oppression story links us with readers who may have faced and experienced similar instances of oppression, thus, building relationships with those whom we may never know. The true power of oppression stories resides in this open invitation to those who read our stories and make a connection.

When we tell our privilege stories, we begin to acknowledge that we have gained from an imbalance distribution of power. For some of us who grew up with a different set of cultural norms, talking about our own privileges may bring about a sense of guilt and shame because we may be judged by our ethnic communities to be overreaching and lauding our success. Therefore, it can be very easy for individuals, especially those of us whose cultural backgrounds emphasize humility and modesty, to hide our privileges because guilt and shame are difficult experiences to deal with. So, the courage it takes to tell privilege narratives by the authors also implies the need to take and accept responsibility in the ecosystem of oppression.

Our Internal Dialogues and Critical Reflections

Making sense of the intersection of our privilege, oppression, and power experiences takes a microscopic lens to our internal processing abilities, as we have frequently reflected on what may seem both uncomfortable and challenging. For all of the authors, it was a journey of external stimulation (i.e., what was said, something happening in their communities, actions taken by others, etc.) translating into internal processing to create awareness and growth. The authors all reflected on how this self-reflection lead to growth as a leader. None of the authors specified a beginning point and an end point for the processing. Instead, it is something that each author will continue to be challenged by and make strides in. Similar to how we in the field of MFT say that cultural awareness and cultural humility are a never-ending process (Fisher-Borne, Cain, & Martin, 2015; Hook, Davis, Owen, & DeBlaere, 2017), understanding our social location and how the intersectionality of our diversity interacts with our professional roles will be a continuous process. The difficult journey comes when we keep challenging our academic position of power, both in action and processing, while our social location keeps changing and evolving.

The internal processes are often the start of an ongoing occurrence. The authors are faced with many internal complexities that they must navigate toward their continued path as a professor, educator, supervisor, and administrator in the field of MFT. Karen processes the multiplicity of social locations as she looks to develop more leadership qualities and empower others to become leaders. In doing so, she had to first reflect on her experiences of power, privilege, and oppression and determine how best to use her experience to best mentor students while leading an MFT program. Before taking action and connecting more with his students and the Black community, Alexander had to conduct more internal work by reflecting on his privileges as an Asian American male before he could empathize with students and connect with the hurting Black community. This was more action-orientated and focused on challenging his perceptions rather than a passive interaction between his experiences of privilege and oppression. Gita mindfully strikes a balance between privilege and humility in her professorial role, one that requires an action perspective to challenge those two areas. Sergio also has to process his identity as a Latino, heterosexual, Christian man, and the points of intersectionality to come from a not-knowing stance and to open himself to new knowledge. Narumi internally processes layers of intersectionality to create visibility and focus on experiences of discomfort. Hao-Min has a constant experience of processing her relationship with her mother to bring about her own personal agency but also crediting it to her built resiliency. She acts to not allow her relationship with her mother be the sole definer of her leadership role with students. Finally, Christie navigates her White privilege and her marginalization as a woman and strikes a balance between advocacy and challenging her privileges before using her position of power to bring about program change. Each author reflected on how the internal dialoguing had to be action-based rather than a passive acknowledgment. The difference here being that to acknowledge and reflect on our experiences may be an initial step, but must be followed by piecing together our stories of power, privilege, and oppression before we could advocate and promote change. This key element must start with ourselves, and each author's story depicted such process.

Using Power and Privilege to Support the Marginalized

All the authors introduce the discourse of power and privilege into our professional narratives and our place within it. We recognize that we have earned credibility within our professional community, and we do not take our professional advantages lightly. All the authors detail how we use our perceptions of privilege and power to increase our effectiveness with the student population, supervisees, or local community, especially the marginalized populations. Specifically, using our positional power, we seek to build an inclusive and fair environment to restore dignity of faculty and students living on the margins, to encourage discussion of intersecting identities, and to openly express their ideas without the fear of being judged or penalized. Additionally, the use of power and privilege is not just limited to the academic level, but instead extends to our local communities.

The MFT professors are not just called to teach, conduct research, and practice clinically, but we are encouraged and expected to be involved in our communities. We are often asked about our communities of interest and how our missions of diversity affect our mental health community. The social responsibility for academic leaders often is an unwritten expectation within our profession, especially for persons from and representing diverse communities, and our authors described this commitment. Sergio integrates his cultural identity into an ongoing responsibility to support and empower his oppressed Latino students. In addition, Sergio's internal processing of his Christian identity and position of power has taken him to a journey as an ally for the LGBTQ communities. Alexander takes the journey to challenge his perceived privileges as an Asian American to connect with and listen to the local Black community who often do not have access to adequate mental health services.

These stories move beyond the limited focus on less privileged students and faculty colleagues of color; they demonstrate connections with other marginalized groups outside our profession and institution. This connection borrows each author's power derived from the status as professors, supervisors, educators, and administrators so that the marginalized communities can gain more visibility and hopefully promote opportunities for change to occur. We hope that each additional connection with communities that are marginalized can build a vision against systemic and structural racism. One might argue that there is added burden with our acquired positional power. Yet, each author has recognized how their social locations, often conflicting, informed their social and professional identities, have inspired them to contribute to the underrepresented. This vision lights a path toward hope—one which we hope our field will continue to embrace.

Going Forward

This book emphasizes the usefulness of intersectionality in capturing the complexities of our stories about discrimination and privilege from differing social locations. It is meaningful to the authors and editors as the topic of leadership from positions of both power and marginalization, in this case, professors and administrators in MFT education, has been little researched nor discussed. I (Alexander) recall the motto from my undergraduate alma mater (the University of Texas at Austin) "What starts here changes the world." By our day to day decisions and actions, these MFT leaders are slowly transforming shared societal beliefs about our leadership positions based on gender, race, ethnicity, education, and occupation. However, we are cognizant of system and structural constraints. We hope our stories can spark more conversations within academia around social location, and how it has contributed to the way we carry out our daily duties and responsibilities.

Implications

Conversations Surrounding Social Location

Administrators, educators, and practitioners should consider conversations surrounding social location from an intersectional lens in order to build spaces that are committed to interrogating how oppressed and privilege identities might intersect in their professional work. Here are questions that were posted to our authors as they began the process of self-reflection on social location, and how their academic positions have been impacted through their social location. It is especially useful for administrators, educators, clinicians, and supervisors who are interested in helping colleagues, students, and clients who seek out the uniqueness of their lived experiences to consider exploring these questions:

1. Defining your social location

   (a) How have your social cultural locations shaped who you are and how you see yourself?
   (b) What is the relationship between your visible identity and your self-identification, and how is this influenced by your cultural context?

2. As a clinician: reflection on social location in your clinical practice

   (a) How have your cultural influences shaped how clients see you?
   (b) How do these influences affect your comfort level in certain groups and your feelings about particular clients?
   (c) What kinds of assumptions are clients likely to make about you based on your visible identity, your sociocultural context, and what you choose to share about yourself?
   (d) How might your areas of privilege affect your work (e.g., your clinical judgments, theoretical preferences, view of clients, beliefs about mental health)?

3. As a clinical supervisor: reflection on social location from a supervisory context

   (a) How do you define and contextualize your social locations in order to understand and resonate fully with what and how your supervisees are struggling with clinical issues?
   (b) How do you meet your supervisees through both differences and commonalities in social contexts?
   (c) What do you do to provide spaces which allow for identifying and altering dynamics of power, privilege, and social oppression?

4. As an educator: reflection on social location in the classroom

   (a) How might your presence in the classroom alter the environment?
   (b) What is invisible to you due to your privilege?
   (c) What is visible to you being a faculty of color?
   (d) How might students respond to you based on your social identities?
   (e) What needs to occur in the curriculum and in the classroom to account for your social location?

5. As an administrator/leader: reflection on social location in administration/ leadership

   (a) How do your social locations influence your belief in your ability to practice leadership?
   (b) How have contextual influences shape your social positions? What implications might those have on the development of your leadership self-efficacy?

(c) Do you consider yourself a leader/administrator from a social location that is rare among leaders/administrators? What kind of challenges do you encounter?

Conversations Surrounding Internal and External Dialogues

One area, which was evident throughout each authors' reflections, was the internal and external dialogues that occurred and will continue to occur. It is through conversations that people are able to socialize, connect, discord, and discuss. We believe that difficult discussions about our own social location needs to be incorporated when discussing issues of power, privilege, and oppression. These types of conversations can occur between faculty members, within the program and university meetings, during clinical supervision, between clinical colleagues, and during community advocacy meetings. While these conversations may not always be the easiest to have, The following articles—Brady, Sawyer, & Herrera, 2016; Hsieh & Seshadri, 2018; Love, Gaynor, & Blessett, 2016; Murray-Johnson, 2019; Sue, 2016—have provided methods on how to conduct those conversations meaningfully. For instance, programs can provide space to "call-in" faculty to have conversation on microaggressions to promote leadership grounded on transparency, conversation, and self-reflection (Hsieh & Seshadri, 2018). Processing the internal dialogues makes the covert overt like retelling stories aloud in a supportive environment.

Conversations Surrounding Actions

As stories are shared throughout these chapters, it is evident that more actions can be done within higher education system to combat prejudices that disadvantage faculty and students. On a student level, challenging the traditional classroom learning standards and infusing the classroom with more experiential exercises, narrative discussions, and difficult dialogues rather than lecture and PowerPoint presentations. In doing so, we remove the limits of a narrow perspective on education, and thereby diversifying the experience to students who do not fit into traditional education methodology. Often in academia, we can fall into the fallacy that there is a "right" or "wrong" way to educate and engage students to make sure they obtain the knowledge. In doing so, we become egocentric and do not take into account how our social location, power, and privilege may have shaped that ideology. Professors should learn how to introduce and engage intersecting social location, power, privileged, and oppressed stories with students at a developmentally appropriate phase of their educational journey by creating an open and safe space.

This same concept can also be applied from an academic leadership position when working with faculty of color, disadvantaged staff members, and when looking at the methodology of curriculum. Working collaboratively with faculty often times can balance the various power dynamics, which may exist within the context of a faculty group. When senior White faculty collaborate on projects, committees, and program design with junior faculty of color, it gives the opportunity for privilege to be shared both on a rank and race level. These types of collaborations give more opportunities and voice to junior faculty of color and promote diverse perspectives. The hope is to foster a program narrative built on balance of privileged and marginalized perspectives, so, an MFT program can actually practice the standards of diversity, multiculturalism, and inclusion that we all preach from within our great programs.

References

Brady, S. R., Sawyer, J. M., & Herrera, S. C. (2016). Preparing social work students to practice in diverse communities through difficult digital dialogues. *Journal of Technology in Human Services, 34*(4), 376–393.

Brown, B. (2012). *Daring greatly: How the courage to be vulnerable transforms the way we live, love, parent, and lead.* New York City, NY: Gotham.

Christensen, T. (2019). Look away: How the social constructionist approach to social problems channels attention away from the marginalized. *The American Sociologist, 50,* 271–289.

Fisher-Borne, M., Cain, J. M., & Martin, S. L. (2015). From mastery to accountability: Cultural humility as an alternative to cultural competence. *Social Work Education, 34*(2), 5–181.

Hook, J. N., Davis, D., Owen, J., & DeBlaere, C. (2017). *Cultural humility: Engaging diverse identities in therapy.* Washington, DC: American Psychological Association.

Hsieh, A. L., & Seshadri, G. (2018). Promoting diversity and multicultural training in higher education: Calling in faculty. In B. Blummer & J. M. Kenton (Eds.), *Promoting diversity and multicultural training in higher education.* Hershey, PA: IGI Global.

Love, J. M., Gaynor, T. S., & Blessett, B. (2016). Facilitating difficult dialogues in the classroom: A pedagogical imperative. *Administrative Theory & Praxis, 38,* 227–233. https://doi.org/10.1080/10841806.2016.1237839.

Murray-Johnson, K. (2019). Engaging self. *Adult Learning, 30*(1), 4–14.

Sue, D. W. (2016). *Race talk and the conspiracy of silence: Understanding and facilitating the difficult dialogues on race.* Hoboken, NJ: John Wiley & Sons.

Index

© Springer Nature Switzerland AG 2021
K. M.-T. Quek, A. L. Hsieh (eds.), *Intersectionality in Family Therapy
Leadership*, AFTA SpringerBriefs in Family Therapy,
https://doi.org/10.1007/978-3-030-67977-4